the aerobics instructor's handbook

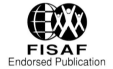
FISAF
Endorsed Publication

Also produced by Network for Fitness Professionals:
The Fitness Leader's Handbook

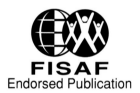

FISAF
Endorsed Publication

The Federation for International Sport, Aerobics and Fitness (FISAF) is an international, independent, democratic, non-profit organisation which is the largest confederation of fitness industry organisations in the world. FISAF members form a synergistic network of expertise, resources and activities. The scope of activity of FISAF and its members includes instructor training and certification, development and production of professional resources, publication of industry journals, and the staging of conventions, expos and sport aerobic championships.

The people who developed FISAF as the world's leading confederation of fitness organisations are Christophe Andanson, Claudio Groso, Volker Ebener, Greg Hurst, Waldyr Soares and Dyanne Ward.

the aerobics instructor's handbook

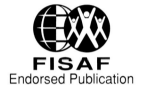
FISAF Endorsed Publication

PRODUCED BY
NIGEL CHAMPION AND GREG HURST
NETWORK FOR FITNESS PROFESSIONALS (AUSTRALIA)

EDITED BY
ANGELEE BOYD, BEd, MEd
LISA CHIVERS, BPE (HONS), MEd

CONTRIBUTORS
LISA CHAMPION, MSc
GREG HURST, DIP PHYS ED, DIP HEALTH ED
CATHY SPENCER, BAppSc

ENDORSED BY
FEDERATION FOR INTERNATIONAL SPORT, AEROBICS AND FITNESS
FÉDÉRATION INTERNATIONALE DES SPORTS, AÉROBICS ET FITNESS

Kangaroo Press

Acknowledgments

The founders of Network for Fitness Professionals — Nigel Champion, Lisa Champion, Greg Hurst and Suzee Miller — extend special thanks to all the dedicated people who have worked for Network in developing outstanding aerobics instructor training: Jeff Ahern, David Allan, Michael Betts, Matt Church, Michelle Dean, Anthea Gilchrist, David Hatch, John Kelly, Sharon Kolkka, Lisa Osborne, Adam Rock, Cathy Spencer, Julie Toyama and Lexie Williams.

For information on membership and activities, please contact Network at PO Box 57, Neutral Bay NSW 2089, Australia. Tel: (61) 02 9908 4944, Fax (61) 02 9908 4349.

AEROBICS INSTRUCTOR'S HANDBOOK

First published in Australia in 1999 by Kangaroo Press
An imprint of Simon & Schuster (Australia) Pty Limited
20 Barcoo Street, East Roseville NSW 2069

A Viacom Company
Sydney New York London Toronto Tokyo Singapore

© Network for Fitness Professionals 1999

All rights reserved. No part of this publication may be reproduced, stored in a retrieval system, or transmitted, in any form or by any means, electronic, mechanical, photocopying, recording or otherwise, without the prior permission of the publisher in writing.

National Library of Australia
Cataloguing in Publication data

Champion, Nigel.
Aerobics instructor's handbook

Bibliography.
Includes index.
ISBN 0 86417 987 1.

1. Aerobic exercises – Handbook, manuals, etc.
2. Physical fitness – Handbook, manuals, etc.
I. Hurst, Greg. II. Title.

613.71

Design by Mega City Publication Design
Cover illustration by Ian Faulkner
Set in 9pt Minion
Printed in Singapore by Kyodo Printing

Contents

Acknowledgments 4

Introduction 6

1 Technical and Instructor Skills 7
Class planning; exercise vocabulary; demonstration;
voice projection; microphone use; instructor positioning;
teaching image; right footing

2 Music 15
Components; music mapping; advantages of the bridge;
music speed and selection; cross-phrasing; sound equipment

3 Base Moves and Elements of Variation 22
Low Impact Aerobics—touch step, step touch, lift steps, march;
High Impact Aerobics; Non-Impact Aerobics; Elements of
variation (DR RT LUMP); armlines; finishing touches

4 Cueing 35
Verbal cueing—What, Where, When, How; non-verbal cueing;
elements of effective cueing; balance of teaching process;
EZQ system

5 Teaching Methodologies 41
Linear progression; pyramid method; add-on method;
link method; holding patterns addition; add and subtract;
layering; organised action; pre-choreography; application
of teaching methods

6 Communication 54
Verbal communication; class introduction; non-verbal
communication; body language and facial expressions;
keys to successful communication; building rapport;
motivation; praise and acknowledgment; education;
handling difficult situations

7 Warm-Ups 64
Integral components; warming the body; mobility;
specific stretching; considerations; specific warm-ups;
methodologies; warm-up concepts

8 Cool-Downs 71
Recovery; flexibility; how to stretch; relaxation; education;
practical applications; special considerations

9 Principles of Muscle Conditioning 78
Myths and misinformation; role of the instructor;
muscle balance; major positional exercises; effective cueing;
key principles

10 Equipment-Based Muscle Conditioning 86
Use of light hand weights and rubberised resistance;
special considerations; exercise vocabulary

11 Step Classes 96
Strengths of Step; stepping safely; the wrong steps;
step heights; music speeds; base moves and Step vocabulary;
muscle-conditioning ideas

12 Class Design and Formats 104
Class descriptions; single- and multi-peak formats; class
grading systems; monitoring intensity levels; timetabling

13 Special Populations 112
The pregnant exerciser; seniors; children

14 Professional Development 118
Qualities of a great instructor; evaluations; participant
expectations; staying motivated; continuing education;
the aerobics co-ordinator; employment issues

15 The Facility 123
Standards and guidelines for the aerobics room and class;
signage; storage of equipment

Appendix I: The Travel Guide 127
Appendix II: Log Book Summary 128
Appendix III: Self-Test 129

Glossary & Bibliography 130

Index 131

Introduction

In recent years a billion-dollar industry has developed from exercising to music, internationally known as 'aerobics'. And with this has grown a great sense of pride and professionalism among aerobics instructors throughout the world, who promote the benefits of this form of exercise. The joy of being able to make an impact on one person or a group of people, their lifestyle choices, health and exercise habits is a real and rewarding experience for an instructor. The energy and adrenaline you feel when leading a highly motivated group of individuals who enjoy exercise to music is truly exhilarating.

But the aerobics instructor's job is not as effortless as it may appear. Few occupations require an individual to put so many skills into practice at once. When teaching aerobics you are required to be a constant motivational force, to deliver a safe and effective workout, to educate and communicate, while still remembering your entire class plan. In addition, you must cue effectively, use the music correctly, and maintain a happy rapport with your participants. And you need to have a high level of physical fitness, so that you appear to be applying all these skills with incredible ease and comfort.

This handbook has been specifically written to provide comprehensive information for new and experienced aerobics instructors, instructor trainers and organisations, aerobics co-ordinators and club managers. It is designed as a text to complement accredited aerobics instructor courses and to bridge the gap between theory and practice. Many examples of the practical application of a range of skills are included, together with drills designed to challenge your understanding of specific aerobics concepts.

Your number one priority should always be to 'know your trade'—this handbook will ensure that you learn all you possibly can about aerobics as a profession. In addition, ever-changing trends require that you keep your mind and attitude open to further learning and professional development.

Be proud to be part of an exciting and dynamic industry. As an aerobics instructor, your dedication to the health, enjoyment and wellbeing of your participants will bring you success and satisfaction.

The Ten Commandments of Aerobics

1. Provide a safe and effective exercise class and abide by industry guidelines.
2. Be a role model for good health, and educate your participants on the benefits of regular exericse and the personal gains they will derive from it.
3. Provide fun and enjoyment for all participants and motivate your class through a variety of techniques and methods.
4. Always stay updated with the latest research and industry trends.
5. Always put your participants' needs first.
6. Set realistic goals for yourself and your participants.
7. Consider differing levels of ability within a class, and cater accordingly.
8. Be prepared for every class you teach, and have confidence in your own ability.
9. Reliably deliver good service to your employer.
10. Set yourself high standards, and always strive to achieve them.

Technical and Instructor Skills

A great instructor is a great teacher. Being an effective aerobics instructor takes much more than performing a series of moves for others to follow. The difference lies in your ability to *teach*, not just lead, and to make that special connection with your class participants. The teaching process must allow your participants to learn and really achieve during your classes. It involves breaking down complex movements to their simplest form and gradually building the finished product. It also incorporates technical information on how to perform exercises correctly. 'Leading' your group involves demonstrating moves with little or no breakdown, and expecting the group to follow. For some instructors, continually breaking down moves and providing technical information may be seen as tedious, but it is the core of what great instructing is all about. Make it your goal to excel as an instructor.

Another important factor to consider is your teaching style, which has a lot to do with your personality and individual style. Many people associate a bubbly, extroverted style as ideal for an aerobics instructor and while this style is popular, many other styles can be equally successful. The most important thing is to be yourself and develop your own unique style. Instructors are individuals and bring a variety of experiences to each and every class. Express your energy and enthusiasm and you will receive these in return.

On your journey into the world of aerobics you will acquire a wide range of teaching skills. Having sound technical and instructor competence involves theoretical understanding as well as the practical application of your knowledge. As an instructor, you will learn to master these skills and continually strive to improve them. You will acquire proficiency in musical interpretation, cueing and communication, exercise selection and choreography development, class design and formats, and evaluation. You will find chapters dedicated to these subjects; additional skills that are crucial to effective instruction are discussed below.

Before proceeding any further, it is recommended that you complete the self-test in Appendix III, which will gauge your knowledge before and after you have completed this handbook. The 'after' results should be a pleasant surprise.

The big picture

Effective instructing incorporates a wide range of skills. As a starting point, consider the following to provide a framework from which all other skills are developed:
- Class planning—the 3 Ms
- Exercise vocabulary
- Demonstration
- Voice projection
- Instructor positioning

The 3 Ms of class planning

Teaching a group for 45 minutes to an hour is certainly a challenge. You need to plan the class from start to finish and, like any exercise session, this includes a warm-up, conditioning phase and cool-down. Having a clear idea of what you want your participants to achieve is important. While class planning incorporates many organisational factors, the three most obvious elements are moves, music and motivation. The 3 Ms are essential for achieving that perfect balance and are discussed below.

M—Moves

You need to select moves and develop choreography that is appropriate for the class in terms of goals and ability levels. In order to be an effective instructor, you need to plan and offer variety to your participants as well as easier and harder options. Every instructor has their favourite moves but variety and a balanced use of muscle groups is important. There may be moves that you don't feel comfortable with but, with rehearsal, you will be able to gradually add these to your repertoire. See Chapters 3 and 11 for Aerobics and Step moves, respectively. In addition to variety, you also need to have good recall to remember your class content. The following methods will assist:

Written notation. Many people enhance their memory by writing their choreography down—this is highly recommended, so that you have record of your previous class. Many instructors feel more confident knowing that these notes are close by even if they do not need to use them during the class. The notes can be placed near the stereo or near your water bottle just in case you need to have a quick glance. If the full set of choreography notes are hard to follow, draw shapes to reflect your travel patterns, or arrows to indicate the travel and direction.

Memorisation. Study and learn your base moves, routines and choreography. Rehearsal is a crucial part of every class. You need to be thoroughly familiar with your choreography and the teaching progression. Practise your choreography to your chosen music; this will assist your confidence and overall teaching ability. If during the class you do forget your moves, put your participants into a holding pattern (a simple move that everyone knows) until you find your place and feel ready to start again.

Class note cards or log books. These are ideal for keeping a record of consecutive classes and, more often than not, an instructor will only change a small portion of the class each time. This is particularly handy when you may not have enough time to prepare for a whole new class. If you keep accurate class logs, these can easily be recycled from time to time. (See Appendix II for a suggested log book format.)

Videos, workshops and master classes. Not only can these inspire you, they also prevent you from getting stale by providing new choreography and teaching techniques. Make your own adjustments on any accompanying notes so that you are able to quickly refer back to these notes.

M—Music

It is usual for the same tape to be played at least a couple of times before using another but, as with moves, variety is important. Avoid using the same tape for months on end. Be sure to cue your tapes to the right spot before the class and always have a back-up tape for those unpredictable situations. When you buy new music, always listen and rehearse to it prior to using it in your class. That way you will be able to use the music to your advantage. See Chapter 2 for further information.

M—Motivation

Be prepared to motivate your group to great heights. Plan for interaction, motivational highlights and social interaction between your participants. When planning for your class, attempt to include at least one form of interaction between your participants. This can include an organised action activity (see Chapter 5), partner exercises or calling out in response to the instructor. Motivation is discussed further in Chapter 6.

Exercise vocabulary

As your skills and experience as an instructor develop, you will have the chance to learn what different moves are called and you will begin to use them with proficiency. Learning the common terms for each move becomes an important part of communication and it is recommended that you make every effort to use industry standardised terms. It is important that all of your centre's aerobics instructors are using the same terminology, to avoid frustration and uncertainty from your participants. Your vocabulary needs to be consistent within a class and from class to class. As your routines develop in classes, you can slightly modify your vocabulary depending on the speed of the combination and participant recall. A common technique is to teach a combination and then give it a name.

The most commonly used lower and upper body terminology is listed in Table 1.1. Prior to examining this table, try the drill below then cross-reference, using the table and Chapters 3 and 11.

Lower body	Upper body
March	Shoulder press
Ezy walk	Chest press
Step touch	Low row
Touch step	Bicep curl
Heels forward	Tricep kickback
Knee lift	Upright row
Leg curl	Lateral raise
Grapevine	Front raise

Table 1.1. **Common exercise vocabulary**

❋ ❋ Drill ❋ ❋

Test your exercise vocabulary. Make a list of all of the base moves you know for a Low Impact class, a Hi-Lo class and a Step class. In addition to this, list all the armlines that you know and the names you have for each of these.

Demonstration

Your demonstration needs to be correct and energetic. Work on your own form and exercise technique, as your participants will use you as a mirror when performing their own exercises. If your technique or form is not correct, your participants' performance will also be incorrect. Instructors will have their own individual movement style and idiosyncrasies. For example, instructors may bend forward at the hips as a way of getting closer to participants and while this is subconscious, it is not a desirable postural position. Movements should be precise, graphic and fluid; avoid being too rigid. Often you will have to adapt your style according to the class. For example, a stronger style may be necessary for muscle conditioning, whereas a dance approach may be appropriate in a Hi-Lo class.

Avoid checking your form and technique in your own classes. Ideally, practise by yourself or with fellow colleagues and use the mirrors to evaluate your form. Alternatively, ask an instructor to watch you, or video yourself for a truly enlightening experience. Always work on increasing your energy and effort levels throughout the class. Remember that participants may only put in approximately 50% of your effort. With this in mind, educate your participants on the benefits of correct technique and form.

Voice projection

An instructor's voice is an extremely valuable tool. Treat your voice with care and never abuse it. Unfortunately there is a high incidence of voice disorders among aerobics instructors, sometimes serious enough to end an instructor's career. Early intervention and good vocal care will help to avoid this occupational hazard.

Although there are different forms of communication used in classes, your voice will always be relied on to educate, instruct, motivate and continually encourage your participants. Every instructor needs to understand how the voice works in addition to employing strategies to preserve their vocal cords and thus protect their livelihood.

How the voice works

The two major bands of muscle that produce sound form the larynx (voice box). The flow of air passing through the lungs causes these cords to vibrate and produce sound. The chest cavities, pockets of the larynx, pharynx, mouth and sinuses can enhance the vibration or resonating sound of the larynx. If any of these cavities become blocked due to illness or other incidentals, then the voice assumes a nasal character.

If you misuse or strain your vocal cords, problems such as voice nodules (pimple-like lumps) or polyps (blister-like lesions) may appear. Don't expect warning signs to appear immediately after you have damaged your voice. In some circumstances conditions such as bilateral voice nodules can go undetected for quite some time.

Warning signs and symptoms of vocal strain can be as simple as a sore or tight throat. Other symptoms may be a raspy or deeper tone to the voice, or a frequent need to clear the throat or cough. A dry or continuous cough may also be a symptom.

Vocal care

- Drink throughout your class to lubricate the vocal cords; always have water close by. Ensure that you are very well hydrated before your class starts.
- If you are teaching back-to-back classes, have a large supply of water and make the effort to drink between classes.
- Warm up your voice, especially if you have a morning class. You may wish to sing or hum quietly to your tapes or to yourself. This will prepare your voice for your class. Allow about five minutes to do this.
- Always keep your cueing and talking clear, concise and to the point. Verbose cueing is a habit that can potentially harm your voice.
- Avoid any type of diuretics (e.g. cola or caffeine) before classes. This will dehydrate the body, including the vocal cords.
- Practise diaphragmatic breathing and project your voice from deep in your abdomen, not from your throat or upper chest.
- Select your music wisely. Females often have trouble being heard over the top of female vocalists or in songs where the pitch in their voices is similar. The same applies for male instructors working with tapes featuring male vocalists.
- Never compromise your voice by using loud music; check your sound levels on a regular basis.

Microphone use

A microphone can be an instructor's best friend or worst enemy. Microphones that do not work properly or are used incorrectly will detract from your class. Every instructor should understand how wireless microphones work and how to use them well.

Microphones are omni-directional and this means that they don't need to be in front of your mouth to pick up your voice. In fact, if the microphone is too close to your mouth, it will pick up and broadcast your breathing and any vocal strain, thus causing distortion. One way to reduce the effects of breathing on the microphone is to use an audio sock or padding over the mouthpiece.

Adjusting the volume to seek good balance between music and voice is a priority when setting up for your classes. For balance to be present between microphone volume and music volume, you must be able to adjust them independently of each other. Always check for feedback. Whilst speaking into the microphone, walk around the room, under the speakers and close to the stereo to identify trouble spots, so that you will know which areas you should avoid during the class.

Never yell or shout into the microphone. The microphone allows you to preserve your voice, so spend time adjusting the volume so there will be no need to shout. The microphone will amplify your normal speaking voice, thus helping to save your vocal cords and making your job much easier.

Headset microphones are best for instructors. Headset fittings vary between different brands of microphones. The headpiece can be moulded to the shape of your head whereas the mouthpiece is much more rigid. You will find three main types of headsets. The first will

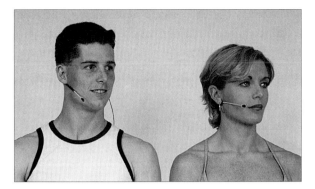

Fig. 1.1. **Microphone headsets**

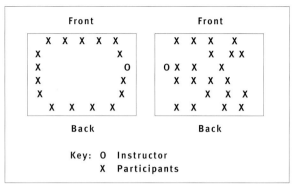

Fig. 1.2. **Two options for instructor-led classes (circle and random)**

have a sliding back that can be adjusted to fit your head; the second will fit over the top of the head; and the third type will fit around the back of the head and loop around the ear. Become familiar with your centre's headset and practise using the microphone correctly so it is both comfortable and an asset to your teaching.

It is quite rare to find hand-held microphones used in fitness centres. If this is the case, ensure that you practise with it before you use it. Such factors as cueing, armlines and routines would also need to be considered. Try to make your statements short, direct and to the point. When holding the microphone, keep the other arm moving and always introduce new armlines slowly, this will give you enough time to cue, demonstrate and participate. Visual previewing can be used for more complicated armlines. Lastly, don't use hand weights when using the hand-held microphone. Not only may you end up with muscle imbalance, you may also lose a few teeth if you try to talk into the hand weight instead of the microphone.

Each centre will have its own system for battery use with the microphone. Some centres request that instructors supply their own batteries and others have their own re-chargeable batteries and a system for use and re-charging.

Instructor positioning

The instructor needs to be visible, but may also need to move around the room to assess participants' form and technique. Don't be afraid to move from the stage or the position at the front of the class. There will be different times during your class when moving around the room is more appropriate than others. The floor work or stretching phases are ideal times for you to move around to correct form and technique. Instructor position will also depend on the class formation as illustrated in Fig. 1.2. A range of formations is covered in Chapter 5 under the heading 'Organised Action'.

In a random formation, it is generally accepted that you face the participants for the majority of the class to maximise voice projection, eye contact and rapport. In smaller studios, facing the mirror may be the only alternative due to a lack of space. You can get eye contact this way but it is not as personal as when you are facing your group. If your choreography involves more complex moves with travel and directional variation, you may need to teach this with your back to the class. When you can see that everyone has mastered the combination, it is recommended that you turn around and face your group. You need to perform this transition smoothly, which requires a good understanding of teaching image and right footing.

Teaching image

The term 'teaching image' refers to the direction the aerobics instructor faces in relation to the participants. The most common images are:

1. **Mirror image** — the instructor faces the participants. The instructor then uses the opposite lead leg to that of the participants and moves/travels as a direct copy or mirror image of the class.

2. **Participant image** — the instructor faces in the same direction as the participants, with his/her back to the participants. The instructor uses the same lead leg as the participants and moves with the class.

Right footing

This is the skill the instructor employs to change teaching image. Participants and instructor perform the same move but the instructor slightly changes the footwork in order to turn around and be leading with the correct leg. The universal trend is for participants to start a move leading with their right foot and the instructor, if in mirror image, will lead on the left foot. Thus, the transition from mirror to participant image will require the instructor to be leading with the right foot, hence the term 'right footing'. However, often the instructor will need to be leading on the left foot, especially when changing from participant image back to mirror image, hence both transitions are important. Remember also, that when you change your teaching image, not only do you need to change lead leg, but the lead arm may also need to be changed.

As an instructor, you need to decide which teaching image is most effective at various stages of your class. The ability to use both images is necessary for two main reasons:

1. To reduce confusion. If a move or pattern cannot be followed, the participants may feel both confusion and frustration. In addition, exercise intensity may decrease and rapport may suffer. Usually, participant image is more suitable for teaching complicated moves and patterns, as participants can more readily follow your foot patterns. Respond to your group quickly and change your teaching image if necessary.

2. Communication and eye contact. Mirror image is accepted as the more effective avenue for developing good communication where eye contact plays an extremely important role. Facing your participants will help build rapport and allow you to make direct eye contact with any participants that may need reassurance or encouragement. Avoid falling in the trap of staying in participant image for long periods of time as your interaction with the group may suffer.

Using both teaching images will greatly enhance your overall teaching ability and make the participants' task of following you an easier one. But, a lot of practice is required to perfect right footing and even the most advanced instructors will continually review their right footing skills in order to teach choreography more effectively. Three methods of right footing follow. Once you have mastered the base moves and feel comfortable working with the music, return to this chapter and try these examples. The figures should assist where the male is the instructor and the female is the participant.

1. Weight variation

This method refers to moves that are either 'weighted' such as a march, or 'unweighted', such as a step touch. In order to right foot, the move must change from a non-weighted to a weighted move or vice versa. Each step in a march is weighted, therefore one of these steps must become unweighted in order to change lead leg while turning around. The footwork for four marches on the spot is 'march, march, march, march'. When right footing, this becomes 'march, tap (while turning around), march, march'. Many marching variations include a tap or knee lift, therefore when right footing the technique may vary.

The touch phase in the step touch is non-weighted and the instructor simply changes this to a weighted step during the turn-around. The footwork for two step touches is 'step, touch, step, touch'. When right footing, it changes to 'step, step (while turning around on the spot then continues with) step, touch'. This method is also used for all step-touch variations.

Sample choreography

Move A = 4 x step touches (8 counts)
Move B = 4 x heel fwd (8 counts)
R = right leg lead
L = left leg lead
* = right footing

Participant
Step touch R, step touch L, step touch R, step touch L
heel R, heel L, heel R, heel L

Instructor
Starts in mirror image—step touch L, step touch R, *
step step L, step touch L.
Now in participant image—heel R, heel L, heel R, heel L.

Therefore, the footwork for an instructor would be: step touch, step touch, step step, step touch. This should be said or cued to yourself when you are learning this method.

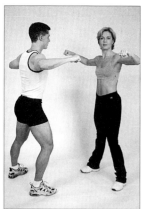

1. Step touch in mirror image
2. Heels forward in participant image

Fig. 1.3. **Right footing—weight variation**

with both feet together on the ground with equal weight bearing on each foot. An example of this may be a star jump, squat or heel raise. By using a neutral footing move that has already been taught as a part of the choreography, an instructor can easily turn from participant image to mirror image or vice versa. The instructor will now be ready to continue with the correct lead leg. Many instructors find it easiest to right foot on a neutral move.

Sample choreography

Move A = 1 x ezy walk (4 counts)
Move B = 2 x jumping jacks (4 counts)
Move C = 4 x alt. step touches (8 counts)
* = right footing
Participant
Ezy walk R, jumping jack, jumping jack, step touch R, step touch L, step touch R, step touch L.
Instructor
Starts in mirror image—ezy walk L, *jumping jack, jumping jack
Now in participant image—step touch R, step touch L, step touch R, step touch L.

2. Repetition variation

This refers to touch steps such as a toe touch side, and lift steps such as a knee lift where changing the number of repetitions allows the instructor to change their image and lead with the correct leg. By repeating the move on the same leg while turning around, a successful transition can be achieved. Instructors need to take care when right footing to ensure that their support leg is not overly stressed. Always try to incorporate a hop to avoid turning on a weight-bearing leg.

Sample choreography

Move A = 4 x alt. knee lifts (8 counts)
Move B = 8 x marches (8 counts)
* = right footing
Participant
Knee lift R, knee lift L, knee lift R, knee lift L
march R, march L, march R, march L, march R, march L, march R, march L.
Instructor
Starts in mirror image—Knee lift L, knee lift R, *knee lift L, knee lift L (i.e. sgl, sgl, dbl).
Now in participant image—March R, march L, march R, march L, march R, march L, march R, march L.

3. Choreographed neutral footing

Neutral footing is best defined as a move that finishes

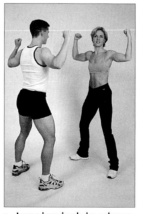 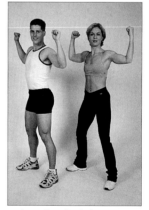

1. Jumping jack in mirror image
2. Jumping jack in participant image

Fig. 1.4. **Right footing—choreographed neutral footing**

These right-footing methods are ideal for a quick and smooth transition from mirror to participant image or vice versa. However, it is also acceptable for the instructor to 'stop, talk and turn'. This is where the instructor establishes a move with the participants, who continue, but the instructor stops to communicate to the group—perhaps a warning of changes to come—then the instructor turns around and joins the class in participant image.

If your participants are not familiar with both images, warn them in the class introduction that you will both face them and move with them. To avoid confusion it may be appropriate to inform the class of this by saying 'Continue, I'm going to join you'.

❊ ❊ Drill ❊ ❊

Once you feel comfortable with the three different right-footing methods, select four moves and construct a simple combination where there is one directional variation and one travelling move. Assuming that you start in mirror image, decide when it would be best to right foot so that the travel and directional variation can be mastered with you in participant image. Then decide on how to return to mirror image once the combination has been mastered.

Music

Music is one of the best things about being an aerobics instructor. It strikes emotions in all of us and often tells a story. Just think of how your favourite song makes you feel. Music has the power to set the scene for your classes. It should compliment the age group of your participants and enhance the mood of both you and your participants. Music can be a major component in the success of any class. It can be used to your advantage in a class setting by inspiring good choreography and by motivating your participants.

The musical requirements of an aerobics instructor are different to those of a musician. Aerobics music must be selected and arranged specifically for exercise. Music terminology and techniques have been developed specifically for aerobics—this chapter will cover the world of music for aerobics instructors.

The components

Music is made up of a series of beats arranged in regular rhythmic patterns. Music is a form of communication and, like any language, it can be powerful when spoken fluently. Like the spoken word, it possesses its own grammar and punctuation. Learn to follow the rules and you can be speaking the universal language of music.

A **beat** can be best described as a musical word, a repetitive pulsing sound of music. It is definite, but can also be underlying. This definite beat is the most easily recognised rhythm or pulse in a song. This is what you will click your fingers or tap your foot to. In aerobics, we want to move with the beat:

1 beat = 1 count

A **phrase** is like a musical sentence. In aerobics, a phrase refers to 8 beats or counts of music:

1 phrase = 8 counts

A strong beat will signify the start of a phrase. When you exercise 'on phrase' you start on beat 1. If you were to change exercises on any other beat, you would be 'off the phrase'.

Phrasing is not always an easy tool to pick up. Some instructors have the ability to understand phrasing much quicker than others. Learning to phrase takes a lot of practice and at first you will really need to concentrate on being able to move in time with the music. Try to master this skill before you start to instruct.

Before examining the phrased choreography example below, it is important first to understand the number of counts it takes to perform a move, and how many repetitions (reps) are in a phrase.

1 march	= 1 count	= 8 reps in a phrase
1 step touch	= 2 counts	= 4 reps in a phrase
1 grapevine	= 4 counts	= 2 reps in a phrase
1 ezy walk	= 4 counts	= 2 reps in a phrase
1 twist	= 1 count	= 8 reps in a phrase
1 knee lift	= 2 counts	= 4 reps in a phrase
1 star jump	= 2 counts	= 4 reps in a phrase

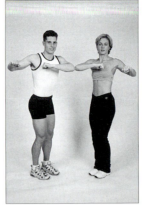

5. Twist

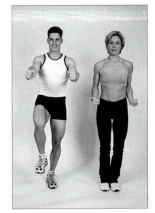

6. Knee lift

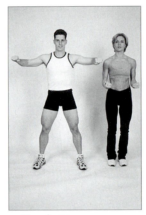

7. Star jump

Fig. 2.1. **Common moves**

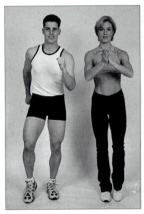

1. March

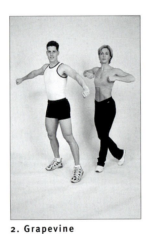

2. Grapevine

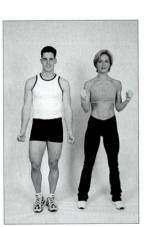

3. Step touch

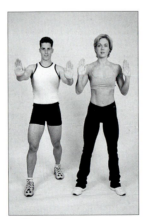

4. Ezy walk

Phrasing for Hi-Lo and Step

Counts	Move	Lower Body	Travel	Direction
Hi-Lo				
1–8	A	2 x grapevine	Lat	Face front
9–16	B	4 x knee lift	OTS	Face front
8 + 8 = 16 phrased				
Step				
1–8	A	2 x alt knee lift R, L	OTS	LDF, RDF
9–16	B	2 x basic step R	OTS	Face front
8 + 8 = 16 phrased				

A **block** is like a musical paragraph and is made up of 4 phrases, or 32 counts. The block is the basic building unit for instructors, providing a framework for creating choreography. Most pre-recorded aerobics music tapes today are produced to work in blocks of 32 counts throughout the 45-minute to 1-hour tape, making your job as an instructor much easier.

1 beat	=	1 count
1 phrase	=	8 counts
1 block	=	32 counts

Listen to your aerobics class tapes in an effort to understand when to start on the first phrase of a block; always listen for the heavy beat. Often there is a distinct change heard at the start of a block. A change in the music will signify the end of a block. Simple drills can be done to learn to understand the music better.

❧ ❧ Drill ❧ ❧

Find yourself a pre-recorded aerobics tape, with an experienced instructor who feels confident with musical phrasing. Listen to your selected music piece and clap your hands on what you think is the first beat of the phrase. An extension of this can be done by putting your hand up at the start of the block. Continue to clap at the start of the phrase (beat 1 of 8) in each of the next 3 phrases within the block.

Professional aerobics music tapes are evenly phrased to make an instructor's job easy. Be careful if you add your own tracks—they may not be phrased. Tapes that are not pre-recorded may not be evenly phrased throughout each song. Such irregularities will require you to change the pattern of your moves to fit the music.

A **bridge** is a musical exception to the rule. The bridge occurs where any group of beats does not complete a block of 32 counts. Bridges provide that sudden musical surprise and the most common form of bridges may be 2 beats, 4 beats, 8 beats, or 16 beats.

Bridges can appear in any part of a song, but usually after the block in the verse, chorus or instrumental. Professional aerobics music tapes will have bridges removed. If you use music with bridges you should pre-choreograph movements to handle the bridge.

Music mapping

In order to teach an aerobics class, the aerobics instructor must first understand the structure of music and be able to construct music maps. Teaching competently to music involves the utilisation of music maps to plan movement sequences and overcome music bridges. The process called *music mapping* is the written breakdown of music into an ordered arrangement of beats that allows you to understand the structure of the song. Knowing the landmarks or parts of a song will assist you in cueing and preparing your participants effectively as a whole. The landmarks of a song include:

Introduction. This is the lead-in for a song, usually building in strength. Songs may simply start as a basic beat and add instruments and voices throughout the introduction.

Instrumental. This can be made up of a number of instruments together or solo. Generally instrumentals follow the melody or tune of the song and commonly appear after the chorus.

Verse. The story of a song, which is generally sung but may be spoken.

Chorus. The musical milestone, repeated often throughout the song to create familiarity.

Pre-chorus. This sits between the verse and chorus. It signals the chorus and is also repeated like the chorus.

Break. The song breaks down to a bare minimum (such as bass beat only). The sound is emptier, and provides a great place to introduce a new song in beat-mixed tapes.

Loop. Just as an introduction signals the start of a song, many songs have a loop to indicate the end. This may be a repeated chorus or a few lines from the chorus. It could be the main melody repeated over and over again at the end of the song. Spotting the repetitive sound will allow you to pick the approaching end of a song.

Mapping the music is easily achieved by creating an

easily followed table (see Table 2.1). To create a music map you need to start with any song that has a catchy beat that you may wish to include in your class. Listen to it a few times to become familiar with it. Draw or copy a table similar to Table 2.1, to include the introduction, the verse, pre-chorus, chorus, instrumental, etc. While listening to the song several times, first try to identify the landmarks in the song and then the phrases.

When recording the phrases, you will need to start recording when you hear the first regular beat. On the first regular beat, it becomes easy to use the stab and drag method. This involves stabbing your pen on the page of the music map on beat 1 and dragging it down to form a line at the conclusion of the eighth count. Do this for all the phrases and watch for any blocks (4 phrases). Write one block per line and try to note the landmarks of the song. Each time you hear a 'change' in the music, move down to the next line, even if a block has not been completed. Any irregularities or bridges in the song should be circled, and you should indicate beside it how many counts that bridge contains.

It is important to note that pre-mixed tapes for aerobics are generally bridge-free. New songs that you may wish to use for a warm-up or cool-down will need to be mapped if you are going to use routines. Linear progression (see Chapter 5) will make it easier for you to handle bridges in warm-ups and cool-downs.

Landmark	I AM WHAT I AM	
	Guide	Map
Intro	beat starts here	////
Verse 1		////
Pre-chorus	and so what	////
Chorus	I am what I am	16*
Verse 2		////
Pre-chorus	melody lifts and builds	////
Chorus	I am what I am	////
Inst	percussion	////
Inst	synth	////
Break/inst	percussion and whooshy sounds	////
Inst	synth	////
Inst	synth	24*
Verse 3		////
Pre-chorus	one life	////
Chorus	I am what I am	12*
Inst	piano	16*
Vocal loop	ooh I am	////
	I am worthy	////
	I am	////
	ooh ooh I am	////
	ah ha	////
Mix	guitar mixing into next song	////
* Bridges		

Table 2.1. **Music map**

Advantages of the bridge

Bridges are not always a disadvantage when planning choreography. All instructors should be able to develop and employ the following strategies to overcome the problem of bridges:

Holding patterns are base moves that everyone knows, such as marching or jogging on the spot. Instructors will hold the group in a simple base move and use a verbal countdown. The verbal countdown will get the group back into their routine after the bridge, or signify a new move to start.

Continuation of last move. When a bridge is coming up in your music, it is very easy to continue the last move in your combination until the bridge is over.

Continuation of first move. By holding your group on the first move of a combination and increasing the repetitions of this move, you can overcome the bridge in the music and prepare your participants to move on. This will reinforce the first move and bring participants back to their starting point. You use this method when you forget the bridge is coming—just act as though you planned it and you will be fine.

Reduce repetitions to complete the entire combination. Knowing a song map well will allow you to reduce the repetitions of your moves to complete the full combination before beginning a new phrase, e.g. 4 reps of each 4 two-count moves will equal 32 counts, 2 reps of each move will equal 16 counts, and this will fill a 16-count bridge.

Introduction of a new move. Complete your existing movement pattern and introduce the new move when the bridge begins. This bridge can be used to commence a whole new movement pattern combination.

Focus point. The bridge may be used for a point of inspiration. Something special or extra can alter the focus of the movement combination. An example of the focus point can be a power option put into the routine to overcome the bridge. The instructor may cue 'jog on the spot and give me all of your energy' and count down to return to the original combination, or insert a movement pattern to reflect the music, e.g. with Latin music, the instructor may insert 3 mambos into the 12-count bridge to give the class a real mood change. Focus points can also be used to increase the intensity or change the mood of the workout. The possibilities are endless—test out your creativity.

✄ ✄ Drill ✄ ✄

Try the methods of using a 16-count bridge to your advantage through the use of the four simple moves below.

Counts	Move	Lower Body	Travel	Direction
1–8	A	4 x alt. heel fwd	OTS	Face front
9–16	B	4 x alt. side touch	OTS	Face front
17–24	C	4 x alt. touch behind	OTS	Face front
25–32	D	4 x alt. knee lifts	OTS	Face front

32 counts = 1 block

Music speed

Music speed plays an important role in determining:
1. how easily your participants can follow and stay in time with the music;
2. their safety in all class formats.

The recommended range of music speeds listed in Table 2.2 are for different class types, and it is suggested that you use this chart regularly. Always check with this chart if you are unsure of the speed for a particular class format.

The bpm, or beats per minute, for each song are generally listed with all aerobic music tapes. However, to find the bpm for each song—if you do not have this information recorded with your tape—time the song for 15 seconds and count every beat, then simply multiply this number by four, just like doing a pulse check. This will now allow you to find the suitability of the music speed to your desired class format.

Class/Component	Recommended Range
Warm-up	130–138 bpm
Low impact	136–148 bpm
Mixed impact (HIA & LIA)	145–165 bpm
Muscle conditioning	70–132 bpm
Interval work	145–165 bpm
X-high intensity	165–185 bpm
Relief	70–145 bpm
Step	118–128 bpm
Cool-down	⟵ 120 bpm

Table 2.2. **Recommended music speeds**

Modern tape decks have a small pitch control button. The pitch control can be used to alter the speed of music. Music speed may be reduced as well as increased.

As an instructor, your role in selecting the correct music speed for your class format and for your participants is a very important one. Don't regard an increase in music speed as a way of increasing intensity. The music speed guidelines have been set for safety and control during your planned workout. Intensity can be achieved by many methods other than by increasing the music speed. You can achieve intensity through the use of propulsions, armlines above the shoulders, and repetition of movement patterns. You must assess your participants throughout the class and make professional decisions based on safety and effectiveness. Remember, as participants become fatigued and music speed increases, the likelihood of injuries can increase.

Increasing music speed

Music speed may be increased only when you are using a tape slightly slower than the recommended bpm range. Music speed can be increased as a motivational tool, providing it is still within the recommended bpm range. To mark the successful completion of a combination by your group in class, you may wish to increase the music speed to perform that combination as a finale during Hi-Lo routines, whilst still remaining in the recommended bpm range.

Decreasing music speed

Music speed may be decreased in situations where you are catering for lower ability, such as the deconditioned or beginners, when teaching and developing combinations in any class, or when using a tape slightly faster than recommended bpm range.

Selection

When selecting your music for class formats, always try to remember the following guidelines:
- Music should always be motivational.
- Music speed should always be the appropriate beat per minute for the type of class.
- A regular beat should be clearly defined.
- Keep within the recommended range of bpm.

Cross-phrasing

A more advanced instructional technique when working with music is termed *cross-phrasing*. Cross-phrasing commences on count 1 but does not continue in regular sets of 8. Due to this inconsistency, it is not recommended for beginners. To identify whether a combination is on phrase or cross-phrased, begin by adding the counts taken for each move or repetitions of each move in sequential order. If, when adding these counts, they amount to 8, and then 16, the sequence is phrased. If they do not add up to 8, but eventually add to 16, the sequence is cross-phrased. Examples for Hi-Lo and Step follow.

Cross-phrasing

Counts	Move	Lower Body	Travel	Direction
Hi-Lo				
1–4	A	Grapevine R	Lat	Face front
5–12	B	4 x knee lift	OTS	Face front
13–16	A	Grapevine L	Lat	Face front
4 + 8 + 4 = 16 cross-phrased				
Step				
1–6	A	1 x two knee repeater R	OTS	Face front
7–12	B	1 x two knee repeater L	OTS	Face front
13–16	C	1 x basic step R	OTS	Face front
6 + 6 + 4 = 16 cross-phrased				

Cross-phrasing rules

Cross-phrasing is a great tool for variety and, to remain manageable, should only last for 16 counts. This is known as the '16 count Cross-phrasing Rule'. Phrasing was designed to provide logical sequences giving a subconscious 'landmark' beat to commence or finish a sequence. It is possible to join two separate 16-count cross-phrased sequences to develop a block (32 counts) of choreography. A creative block of choreography will develop while still maintaining the essential landmark beats.

Cross-phrasing can be developed by two methods:

1. Grouping and dividing

A combination may consist of two moves (ie. Move A and Move B). By grouping the repetitions of Move A and then grouping the repetitions of Move B together, the combination will be in its simplest form, e.g. A+B. By dividing the repetitions of one of the groups, the combination can become cross-phrased and more challenging, e.g. half of A, all of B, then the other half of A (see Hi-Lo example above).

2. Irregular repetition

Cross-phrasing can be easily created by using irregular repetitions of moves. The counts taken for these irregular repetitions need to be balanced to satisfy the 16-count Cross-phrasing Rule (see Step example above).

Cross-phrasing is a teaching tool that can give your classes that extra sparkle, providing you are prepared for it. If it is not used successfully, with correct cueing and preparation, it can be equally disastrous. Cross-phrasing should be used sparingly and the majority of your class should be phrased. Work out your sequences correctly before attempting to cross-phrase. Learn your moves first and then learn your cueing to fit the moves.

Sound equipment

As an instructor you will not only be taught to select suitable exercises for the various segments of a class, and for different class formats but, because music plays such a vital role in planning your classes, it is also essential that you acquire skills in the purchasing and storing of aerobics tapes and the correct use of sound equipment.

Ensure that you familiarise yourself with all elements of sound operations in your fitness centre. Check the basic power connections and know the controls on the system that affect the sound. Always balance your treble and bass. Treble is the top of the sound spectrum and bass is the low-pitched beat. Walk around the room and test out the effects treble and bass have on your tapes. Quite often the sound is projected out towards the participants, so don't be afraid to test out your sound before and during your class. Move around the room and feel the effect the music has at different points in the room. Learn to balance both your music and voice levels.

If you work in only one fitness centre, then maintenance of your sound system is of vital importance. Always clean heads and rollers on the deck after every 10 hours of usage. De-magnetise heads at regular intervals, as tapes can be erased with magnetic field build-up. Magnets located inside speakers can erase tapes, so avoid leaving your tapes on the speakers.

Always close the cassette deck tape insertion door after use to keep the inside dust-free, and check leads and extensions routinely. If you are a freelance or part-time instructor, always check that the centre maintains the system, in order to protect your own investment in tapes and equipment.

Specialised aerobic music tapes are a definite benefit to the industry. In order to get maximum life out of your tapes, always store them in their individual cases away from magnetic fields, heat and moisture. Never leave your tapes in the car during the heat of the day.

You will eventually build a big library of aerobic music tapes which will allow you to rotate your music for classes. Just in case something does go wrong with the sound system or your tape, ensure that your are always prepared and that you carry a spare tape with you whenever you teach classes.

Ensure that you listen to newly purchased tapes before you attempt to use them in a class. This will help you to avoid the 'Oops, I didn't know that was there' or 'Sorry, this is a new tape' syndromes. If you have new tapes that do have bridges throughout the songs, map these tapes for your own regular referral—this will enhance the effectiveness of your planning and teaching. Most new pre-recorded tapes indicate that the tapes are bridge-free; always check for this when purchasing aerobic music.

Be aware of the music copyright regulations. Your local instructor organisation should be able to provide you with the relevant information. It is unprofessional and illegal to copy or pirate tapes. Pirating tapes reduces the quality of sound reproduction and ultimately serves to increase the costs for everyone in our industry.

Base Moves and Elements of Variation

Moves are the basic building blocks of every aerobics program. The ability to classify base moves and then add variety by applying elements of variation is the first step towards designing a professional class. Creative choreography may easily emerge from the simplest of base moves.

All aerobic moves can be classified into categories. When the moves are broken down into their purest form, we are able to see that there are three main classifications: Low Impact Aerobics (LIA), High Impact Aerobics (HIA) and Non-Impact Aerobics.

Low Impact Aerobics (LIA)

LIA can be defined as movements where one foot is in contact with the ground at all times. Low impact moves are used in the warm-up, cardiovascular, and aerobic cool-down sections of the class. Less impact and stress is placed on the body, as there is no airborne phase—when both feet are lifted off the ground, the impact transmitted to the lower leg on landing is high. The basic principle of a low or light impact move is to reduce the impact caused in jumps, kicks and runs by keeping one foot on the ground at all times. In many instances this will reduce the intensity, which can be counterbalanced by flexing and extending the supporting leg.

The four base categories of LIA moves are:
1. Touch step;
2. Step touch;
3. Lift steps;
4. March.

Special considerations for LIA

Excessive bending of the knee of the supporting leg, and forward trunk flexion, have been used to maintain a high workload, but this may lead to a different range of injuries than is caused in high impact exercise. The back should normally be kept vertical and if a move requires forward flexion, 10–15 degrees is usually enough; even this should not be maintained for long periods.

Ensure that the supporting leg remains slightly bent and the trunk is not flexed too far forward. Keep the shoulders and head up.

1. Touch step

This is where the toe or heel is moved away from the supporting leg, touches the floor, then is returned to the starting position and steps together, i.e. touch then step. This category includes toe touches (or taps) to the side, behind and in front, and heels forward and to the side. Always start in a narrow stance, feet together.

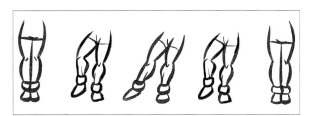

Fig. 3.1. **Toe touch side**

Description: Keep the supporting leg bent and touch the toe of the opposite leg on the floor to the side.

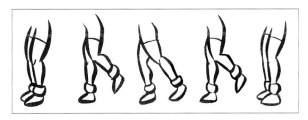

Fig. 3.2. **Toe touch behind**

Description: Keep the supporting leg bent and push the toe of the opposite leg directly behind onto the floor. Do not push the heel down.

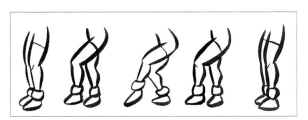

Fig. 3.3. **Toe touch front**

Description: Keep the supporting leg bent and push the toe of the opposite leg in front of the body onto the floor.

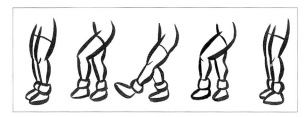

Fig. 3.4. **Heels fwd**

Description: Keep the supporting leg bent and push the heel of the opposite leg forward onto the floor.

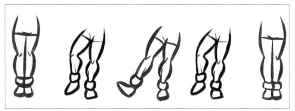

Fig. 3.5. **Heels side**

Description: Keep the supporting leg bent and push the heel of the opposite leg to the side onto the floor.

2. Step touch

This base move involves stepping out laterally (sideways), then touching the toe of the trail leg lightly on the floor so you can step immediately in the opposite direction, i.e. right then left. The 'touch' can be changed to a heel, leg curl or knee raise, but you always step first.

Description: With the legs together, start the move by

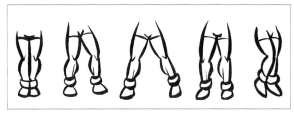

Fig. 3.6. **Step touch**

stepping out laterally and transfer the body weight onto this leg. Bring the other leg over and touch lightly on the floor. Repeat this move with the other leg to return to the starting position.

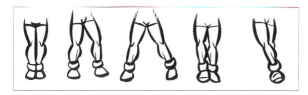

Fig. 3.7. **Step heel**

Description: Step out laterally and instead of touching the floor with the toe of the trail leg, place the heel down in place to create a wide stance, by crossing the heel in front of the lead leg.

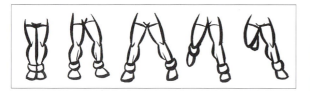

Fig. 3.8. **Step curl**

Description: Step out laterally, then bring the heel of the trail leg towards the buttocks.

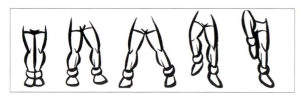

Fig. 3.9. **Step knee**

Description: Step out laterally, then pull the knee of the other leg up in front of the body, flexing the knee and the hip during the lift.

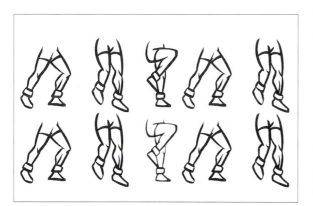

Fig. 3.10. **Step knee repeater**

Description: As in the step knee, the knee repeater involves lifting the knee but in repetitions of 2, 3 or 4 to fit in with the music.

Special considerations: Perform no more than 8 consecutive knee repeaters on one leg to avoid repetitive foot strike patterns. Ensure that working leg is tapped lightly on the floor between knee lifts.

Variations

Another variation of the step touch is the double step touch which, as the name implies, consists of two steps to the side. A grapevine is a variation of the double step touch.

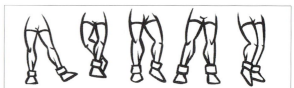

Fig. 3.11. **Grapevine**

Description: In the grapevine, the trail leg crosses behind the supporting leg when performing the double step touch. The grapevine is cued by simply saying: 'step, behind, step, together'. The leg can also be crossed in front of the supporting leg during the grapevine. A double grapevine can be performed by bringing both legs together with a small jump between grapevines, or by stepping the leg in front in between the two grapevines. Legs will then go behind, in front and behind for the double grapevine.

3. Lift steps

This category of moves involves a lifting action such as a knee lift, kick, side leg lift and leg curl.

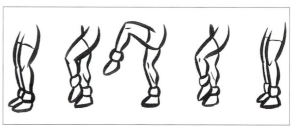

Fig. 3.12. **Knee lift**

Description: Keep the supporting leg bent and lift the knee of the opposite leg. The knee is bent and lifts straight towards the chest. The lifted leg is than lowered and the move is repeated on the opposite leg.

Special considerations: The bent leg shortens the lever, making it slightly easier and also safer. Avoid leaning forwards.

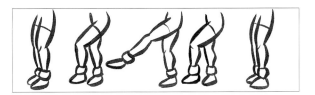

Fig. 3.13. **Kick**

Description: Keep the supporting leg bent and lift the opposite leg in front. The lifted leg is straight, with a very slight bend to avoid locking at the knee joint.

Special considerations: In most situations the leg need only be lifted to approximately 45 degrees. Too much emphasis is often placed on kicking the leg as high as possible, but this can cause poor spinal alignment and/or a ballistic effect, leading to hamstring strain.

The bottom leg must stay slightly flexed and the heel kept on the floor. The back should be upright and the head facing forward.

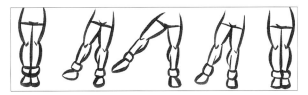

Fig. 3.14. **Side leg lift**

Description: Keep the supporting leg bent and lift the opposite leg out to the side. The lifted leg is straight, with a very slight bend in the knee.

Special considerations: The leg does not have to be lifted high to the side. Keep the movement low and controlled to maintain body alignment and form.

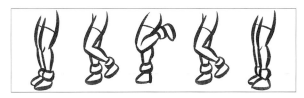

Fig. 3.15. **Leg curl**

Description: Keep the supporting leg bent and curl the opposite leg behind the body, bringing the heel towards the buttocks.

4. March

Marching (or walking) is a common, familiar move used throughout aerobics choreography and as a holding pattern. Variations include walking forwards/backwards (fwd/bwd), V-steps or Ezy walks, and marching out and in.

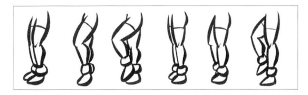

Fig. 3.16. **March OTS**

Description: Simply march or walk lifting one leg at a time on the spot (OTS). Natural arm movements can accompany the march.

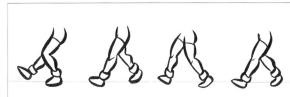

Fig. 3.17. **Walk fwd/bwd touch**

Description: Start the travelling move by walking forwards for 3 counts (large steps). On the fourth count, bend the supporting leg and touch the toe or heel of the forward leg onto the floor, i.e. walk, 2, 3, touch. Repeat the move backwards.

Special considerations: Be sure to prepare participants for a forward to a backward movement, or a backward to a forward movement.

base moves and elements of variation

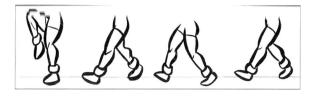

Fig. 3.18. **Walk fwd/bwd knee lift**

Description: As for Figure 3.17, but instead of touching the floor, lift the knee of the forward leg on the fourth count, i.e. walk, 2, 3, knee. Repeat backwards.

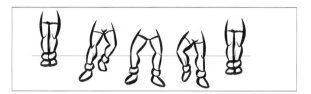

Fig. 3.19. **V-step or ezy walk**

Description: Start with legs together and step one leg in front and wide and then the other leg, to create a V-shape with legs apart in a wide stance. Complete the movement by stepping the first leg back to its original position and then the other left so that the feet are now together again. The move can be cued as: fwd, fwd, back together, or wide, wide, back together.

Special considerations: Ensure the feet go from a narrow stance to a wide stance and back together to a narrow stance.

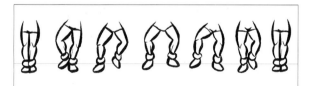

Fig. 3.20. **March out and in**

Description: Starting with feet together, take one foot at a time out to each side to create a wide stance, then march the legs back together, i.e. out out, in in.

High Impact Aerobics (HIA)

HIA is defined as a movement that has an airborne phase, i.e. both feet may be off the ground at the same time. This airborne phase creates considerably more force or impact to the body than do low impact moves.

The four base categories of HIA moves are:
1. Jumping;
2. Lift jump/hop;
3. Step jump/hop;
4. Jogging.

1. Jumping

Jumping is a compound exercise that quickly elevates the heart rate. This is where both feet lift off the floor and land at the same time. Examples include jumping jacks, squat jump, squat jack, ski jump and jump fwd/bwd.

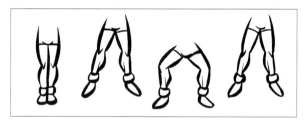

Fig. 3.21. **Jumping jack**

Description: Start with feet together and hands by the side. Jump the feet to shoulder width apart. Flex at the ankle and knee joint upon landing to absorb the impact and ensure that the knees are in line with the feet.

Special considerations: Do not spread the legs too wide when jumping. This can stress the knee joint and cause pelvic floor and uterine ligament problems in women.

Be cautious in swinging straight arms in a full arch from the sides to above the head. If this is done, allow more time for each movement and do not keep the hands facing out, as this may stress the shoulder joint. Turn palms to face forward to relax the shoulders. The jumping jack is a safer alternative to the traditional star jump.

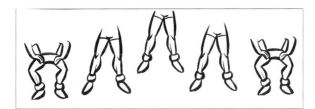

Fig. 3.22. **Squat jump**

Description: Stand with feet comfortably apart, knees bent to a quarter squat. Jump high, reach up with hands, then land with feet comfortably apart. On landing, absorb the impact in the ankles and knees by landing softly and bring the hands down to the knees for support. This can be further varied by pushing one arm up and then the other.
Special considerations: Do not bend the knees to an angle less than 90 degrees and do not touch the ground with the hands.

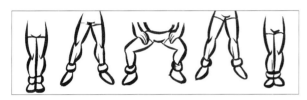

Fig. 3.23. **Squat jack**

Description: Stand with feet together. Bend the knees and perform a jumping jack but land in a squat position with the knees bent, feet wide and toes slightly turned out. Push off from this wide stance to jump up and bring legs back together.
Special considerations: Keep the knees soft at all times.

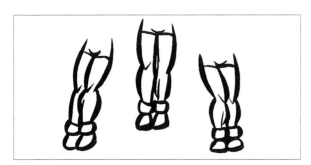

Fig. 3.24. **Ski jump**

Description: Start with feet comfortably apart, bend knees and jump to one side. Keep knees bent on landing, then push off and jump to the other side. Speed of the movement can vary from fast to slow.
Special considerations: Keep knees bent at all times to lower centre of gravity to increase stability and support. The jump to each side should not be too wide, as this may cause lower leg injury.

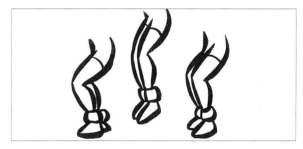

Fig. 3.25. **Jump fwd/bwd**

Description: As in the ski jump, this is a double-legged jump, but the body is now moving forwards and backwards instead of sideways.

2. Lift jump/hop

These moderate to high intensity aerobic moves are the high impact version of the low impact lift moves. A jump or hop is added to actions such as the knee lift, leg curl and kick.

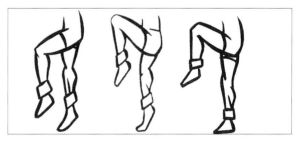

Fig. 3.26. **Knee lift**

Description: Start with feet slightly apart and lift one knee up in front of the body. The supporting leg hops as the knee is lifted and then the feet jump together to change legs.
Special considerations: Ensure a soft knee on the supporting leg and avoid lowering the chest to meet the knee.
Variations: Opposite knee to elbow.

base moves and elements of variation

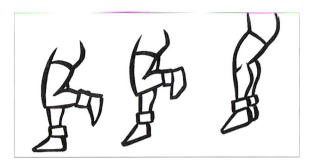

Fig. 3.27. **Leg curl**

Description: Lift one heel towards the buttocks by flexing the knee, then lower the leg. The supporting leg hops as the leg is curled, then the feet jump together to change legs.
Special considerations: Ensure knees remain soft when hopping or jumping. Avoid arching the lower back.
Variations: Opposite hand to heel behind back.

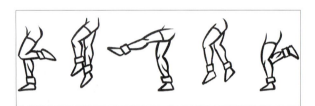

Fig. 3.28. **Flick front**

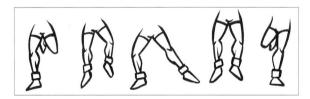

Fig. 3.29. **Flick side**

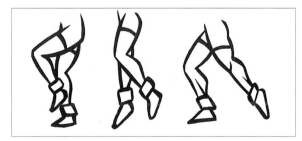

Fig. 3.30. **Flick back**

Description: High impact kicks are commonly known as flick kicks, which can be performed to the front, side or back. These are similar to the standard kick, except that the feet do not come together between kicks. As one leg is lowered, the other leg prepares for the next kick by bending at the knee. The knee is brought forward and the leg performs the flick kick while the supporting leg hops.

3. Step jump/hop

The step touch and its many variations can be performed as a high impact move by adding a jump (e.g. step jump) or a hop (e.g. step knee and step curl).

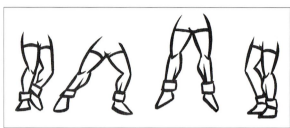

Fig. 3.31. **Step jump**

Description: The step jump is a high impact version of the step touch. Instead of touching the toe to complete the step touch, both legs are brought together with a jump.
Special considerations: Keep both knees bent throughout the move, especially when jumping. Ensure that the body does not rotate, and try to keep the hips and shoulders to the front to allow for an easy change of direction.

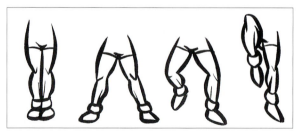

Fig. 3.32. **Step knee**

Description: Start with the legs together and step laterally, transferring the body weight onto this leg. Pull the knee of the other leg up in front of the body. As the knee lifts, the supporting leg hops.
Special considerations: Keep knees soft to absorb the impact.

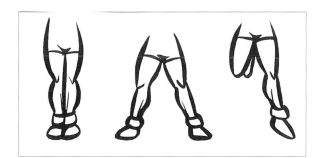

Fig. 3.33. **Step curl**

Description: Start with legs together and step laterally, transferring the body weight onto this leg. Curl the leg of the other leg behind the body, pulling the heel towards the buttocks. As the leg curls to the highest point, the support leg hops.
Special considerations: Keep the knees soft to absorb the impact.

4. Jogging

Jogging is the high impact version of walking and is a moderate to high intensity aerobic move. Variations include the jogging V-step and the pony.

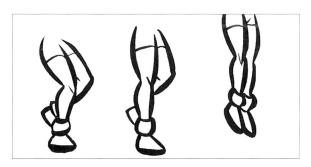

Fig. 3.34. **Jogging**

Description: A 'single' jog is the natural action of jogging. Arms should be swinging naturally in opposition. A 'double' jog incorporates a little hop prior to changing legs. It is also known as a 'double time' jog.
Special considerations: Attempt to ground the heel of the supporting leg and keep the knees slightly flexed.
Variations: Knees up or heels to buttocks.

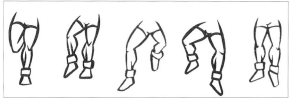

Fig. 3.35. **Jogging V-step**

Description: Jog one leg forward and wide from the narrow starting position. Jog the opposite leg forward and out to complete the wide stance. From this wide stance jog the legs one at a time back to the starting position. This is the high impact version of the ezy walk or V-step.
Special considerations: Keep the knees bent at all times and be prepared to change from a forward to a backward movement.

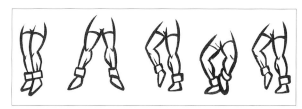

Fig. 3.36. **Pony**

Description: This is a two-count move that can be performed forwards, backwards or laterally. From a regular jog, change the rhythm from 1, 2 to 1 and 2. The lateral pony involves a jog or leap to the side, then two jogs in place, and this is often taught from a step touch.
Special considerations: Keep the movement from side to side quite small, whereas the forwards pony can be large. Take care when performing backwards.

Non-Impact Aerobics

While these moves are usually performed in muscle conditioning, they can be used sparingly in aerobic sections such as the warm-up and cool-down.
  The base moves are:
  1. Lunge;
  2. Squat.

base moves and elements of variation

1. Lunge

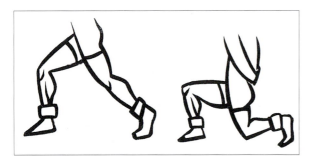

Fig. 3.37. **Lunge**

Description: Stand with one foot in front of the other. Feet should be in line with hips and toes facing forward. Bend both knees and lower towards the ground. Straighten legs and repeat.

Special considerations: Weight should be centred between both legs. When the lunge is taking place, ensure the knee and ankle of the front leg are in line, and no less than 90 degrees should be formed at the front knee. Keep head up and back vertical.

Variations: Alternate lunges—Start with feet together and lunge forwards then backwards, one leg at a time.

2. Squat

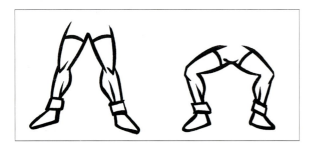

Fig. 3.38. **Wide squat**

Description: The two main foot positions are mid-stance, where the feet are placed shoulder width, and wide, which allows a much wider base of support. It is imperative that the knee joint tracks properly. The knee is designed to flex and extend only in a straight line. As a general rule the knee will bend in the same direction as the foot is pointing. For most people a good squat stance is with the feet turned out anywhere from 10–45 degrees, therefore the knees will bend out over the foot at the same angle.

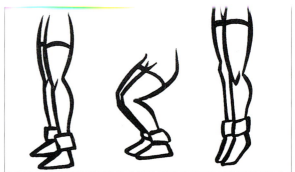

Fig. 3.39. **Squat press**

Variations: A variation is the squat press. Stand with feet in line with hips, feet facing forward and knees bent. Squat, then lift onto toes, straightening the legs as you lift up. Lower down and repeat.

Special considerations: The deeper the squat the higher the load. For a warm-up or for beginners, only use a quarter squat (knee joints bend to approximately 135 degrees). A half squat (100 degrees) is used for a stronger workout, particularly for intermediate and advanced exercisers.

There is a tendency for the knees to roll inwards or to wobble during the squatting movement. This is mainly attributed to weak vastus medialis (inner quad muscles), and can lead to injuries. Encourage correct knee alignment.

The elements of variation

Numerous variations can be derived from these base moves by simply adding the Elements of Variation. It is time to introduce you to the acronym DR RT LUMP to describe:

D—Direction—refers to a change in relation to your body's reference point. Moves can be varied by changing the direction the body faces, e.g. front, back, left and right sides (see Table 3.1). Direction can be cued as 'Turn your jumping jack to the right side, to the back, to the left side and back to the front'. This type of change in direction refers to a rotational change in direction.

1. Front	6. RDB (right diagonal back)
2. Back	7. LDF (left diagonal front)
3. Right side	8. LDB (left diagonal back)
4. Left side	9. Clockwise (rotation–¼, ½ and full circles)
5. RDF (right diagonal front)	10. Anticlockwise (rotation–¼, ½ and full circles)

Table 3.1. **Directional reference points**

R — Rhythm — can be defined as a focus on the up or down beat of the music, or a change of movement speed. This can be done by halving or doubling the amount of time spent on a move, e.g. regular jacks followed by a slower jack. The aerobic style can also emphasise a change in rhythm, e.g. funk classes generally use a rhythm count or cue as follows: and 1 and 2 and 3 and 4, whereas regular classes use a normal rhythm of 1, 2, 3, 4.

R — Repetition — refers to changing the number of repetitions performed on one side of the body before changing to the other side. This includes single, single, double patterns and repeater variations.

T — Travel — refers to moving your body off the spot (see Table 3.2). It is important to define the difference between direction and travel. Quite simply, we can change direction without travelling and we can travel without changing direction. An example of this would be a double grapevine, which faces the front but travels laterally. The Travel Guide in Appendix I details the most appropriate travel patterns for common base moves.

L — Lever — refers to a change in arm and leg length. Changes in arm length can involve changing a long lever lateral raise to a short lever lateral raise. A change in leg length can be shown as a change from a knee lift to a straight kick. An increase in lever length can increase intensity and vice versa.

U — Unilateral/bilateral — Unilateral is where one arm or leg moves at a time, and bilateral is where both arms or legs move at once. A unilateral/bilateral arm pattern would be 2 bicep curls on the right arm, 2 bicep curls left, then 4 bicep curls using both arms. A similar pattern for the legs would be 2 side touches right leg, 2 side touches left, then 4 jacks.

M — Mode — refers to the level of impact, either non-impact, low impact or high impact. Each level of impact can be used to change the intensity of a move.

P — Plane — refers to the physical parameter in which our arms and legs can work, e.g. anterior, posterior, sagittal and transverse plane, etc. Simply, it refers to the direction of our arms and legs. An example of three changes in plane can be shown as: 1. toe touch front; 2. toe touch side; and 3. toe touch behind.

TRAVEL

Travelling: The way in which the body moves towards the directional reference point.

1. Forward (fwd) — the front of the body moves towards the reference point. Remember the difference between the front and fwd. You can travel fwd to the front and bwd to the front of the room.
2. Backward (bwd) — the back of the body is moving towards the directional reference point.
3. Lateral (lat) — the side of the body is moving towards the directional reference point. You can also travel laterally to the front.
4. On the spot (OTS) — the body moves, but either stays or returns within 4 counts to its original starting position.
5. Rotational (rotn) — the body rotates around its central axis. Rotation often involves a combination of forward, backward and lateral travel. Rotation can be done on the spot or towards a directional reference point. Turns of 360 degrees can be made up of 4 x 90-degree or 2 x 180-degree turns. Please note a full 360-degree turn in one move (1 or 2 counts) is considered potentially dangerous and should be avoided. With all rotational travel it is vital to ensure no body part experiences unnecessary stress. It is the responsibility of the instructor to choose safe rotational moves and conditions (ie. enough counts to perform the turn safely, correct music speed and correct cueing methods).

Table 3.2. **Travel**

When cueing for both direction and travel within your class, ensure that you give participants a clear reference point to work towards or away from. This is referred to as the directional reference point. When travelling around your aerobics room, you may also have many landmarks to use as directional reference points including the weight area, the water cooler, the mirrors, the stage or even the equipment

The aerobics room compass in Fig. 3.40 represents the fixed directions for participants in relation to the instructor's home base. This frame of reference should be used at all times when structuring your classes. Further to these directions, when planning for more advanced choreography, a basic 'shape system' can be used as an additional planning consideration or element of variation.

Shape systems refers to the pattern that each participant travels in or traces during their movement sequence. Selected shapes could be as simple as an 'L', 'square', 'circle', 'triangle' or 'cross'. An extension of these shapes can then be labelled as a lettering system, using such letters as M, V, X, U, T or S. Combinations can be written in a basic form and then direction and travel patterns can be added to select the shape of choice. Or you can first draw the shape and then design choreography to fit the shape.

From a teaching perspective, the choreography must be learnt in a basic form before you add direction changes. After the combination has been learnt, when using and cueing the shape system, the cueing can then be set up to directly reflect the shape of the choreography, e.g. '4, 3, 2, L-shape' or '4, 3, 2, T-shape'.

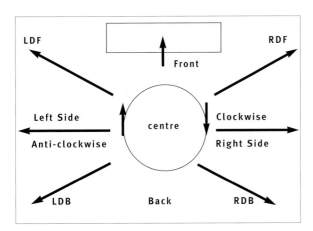

Fig. 3.40. **The aerobics room compass**

When setting up or using your aerobic compass or shape system, special considerations need to be made. These considerations include both the size and shape of your aerobics room. Does it have many pillars or poles in the centre of it? Is it long and thin or very square? Some shapes will be better employed in various room sizes. Ensure that you try out the shapes at many different points in the room in order to get a feel of how your participants will feel completing the shape. Your choreography may need to be simpler when using so many direction and travel patterns. The experience level and number of participants in your class will also play a part in choreography design and planning.

Learn your base moves first, then add direction and travel. Now learn your cueing to reflect each stage of the learning process. You must learn both of these important factors before you attempt to use shapes or new travel and direction patterns. The use of a microphone will bring further ease to this challenge. The microphone will allow your cues to be clear, so keep them as concise and as accurate as possible. Make sure you cue the geographical landmarks or directions early to ensure participants ease and success.

Changing the orientation of your participants during your classes may require you to move around the room as you create your combination. Ensure that you place yourself in the most effective, visible teaching position. To make the participants' workout easier, add a good balance of holding patterns, a balance of intensity to keep the energy in the workout, neutral footing moves that bring both legs back together to establish orientation, and new lead legs and rotational moves so that the combination or shape will be easy to complete.

✗ ✗ Drill ✗ ✗

Work through each category of the low impact moves and apply DR RT LUMP to each move. You should be able to create endless variations. Add these to your exercise vocabulary.

Choreography breakdown

A rule for teaching is, if you cannot break down and teach a combination 'bit by bit', then don't use it. When observing another instructor's class, a video or workshop, it is important that you examine the finished product and try to break it down to its simplest form. What teaching methods were used, how did they cue the changes, how did the participants respond? No combination is worth teaching unless you know how to break it down in order to build gradually and logically. It is important that you do actually teach it and not just demonstrate. The elements of variation can be used to break down more complex sequences and help you to identify the changes that have been made.

As your instructing skills develop, this ability to identify the base moves and elements of variation will certainly allow you to add more variety to routines. It will also allow you to get more mileage out of your existing routines.

Armlines

It is a common practice to offer armlines once participants have mastered the lower body moves. Armlines offer variety and intensity to the workout and can be used to add that special finishing touch to any basic movement pattern. Armlines should not confuse your participants, but rather add enjoyment and a challenge. A simple rule for all instructors to follow when designing their classes should be:

Simple leg patterns: challenging arms.
Challenging leg patterns: simple arms.

Not all armlines will flow from one to the next. Careful consideration should be made when choosing armlines to ensure that the transitions are smooth, especially if hand-held weights are being used. The speed between various arm positions will be affected by the use of hand-held weights, and safety needs to be a prime factor. Determining the starting/finishing position for arms in your combinations does several things: it allows for smooth transitions, and a logical start and finish point for all armlines. The rule of thumb is to ensure the starting position matches the finishing position of the previous armline. This eliminates lever problems that occur with a change in start positions during combinations. It also eliminates some of the confusion felt by participants when trying to cope with a number of start positions within the one combination.

A focus point will ensure that participants maintain good form and control. Armlines can be taught with slower music during the warm-up phase of the class, then the instructor can make use of patterns already taught.

Armlines can be performed in a variety of ways, as follows:

Complementary—armlines follow the direction of the lower body, such as if the body travels laterally, the armlines are also moved in a lateral plane. An example of this may be a grapevine right and left and the armline is a lateral raise, or walking fwd and bwd and the arms are in a low row moving fwd/bwd.

Opposing—armlines oppose the lower body or are performed in a different plane. For example, performing a lateral raise when walking fwd/bwd.

Bilateral—both arms do the same thing at same time (double), hence are symmetrical or balanced.

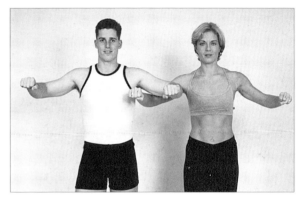

Fig. 3.41 **Bilateral armlines**

Unilateral—only one arm moves at a time (single). For example, 2 bicep curls on the right arm on a grapevine to the right, and vice versa.

Alternating—when one arm follows the other in turn and performs the same armline. For example, bicep curl right, left continuously when walking OTS (Fig. 3.42).

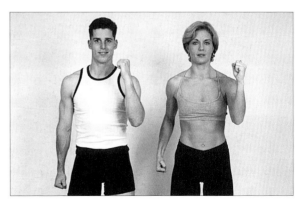

Fig. 3.42. **Alternating armlines**

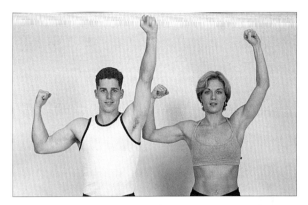

Fig. 3.43. **Asymmetrical armlines**

Asymmetrical —where one arm performs a different armline to the other at the same time (Fig. 3.43).

A more challenging armline is when any of the above variables are combined in a 4-, 8- or 16-count pattern.

Finishing touches

Adding additional flair or flavour to your movement patterns can be achieved by the choice of hand positions to complement your armlines. The four main hand positions are blade, fist, jazz and dance.

Mix and match patterns

After a new arm pattern has been taught, it is possible to achieve maximum mileage out of this by combining a variety of leg and movement patterns. To ensure that success is achieved here, leg or armlines should be automated, i.e. participants must have learnt it and be able to perform it easily. Accent or rhythm changes in the arms must also be compatible with the added arm movement. It is also useful to have a stable or similar part of the combination that does not change, so that your participants can have a mental time-out. The workout should be a physical challenge rather than a mental challenge.

Emphasising the beat

Syncopation can be added to leg and arm patterns to create variety and emphasis on certain musical counts. An example of this could be clapping a 1-2, 1-2-3 pattern. With simple arms, the leg patterns could also adopt a syncopated step, e.g. march, march (1, 2), pony (3 and 4).

Conclusion

In summary, ensure that you use a variety of armlines so that your workouts do not become predictable. Table 3.3 lists common armlines.

Bicep curl	Tricep kickback
Lateral raise	Front raise
Low row	Upright row
Chest press	Pec dec
Shoulder press	Lat pulldown
Punch	Reach
Scoop	Circle
Swing	Criss-cross
Diamond	L-arms

Table 3.3. **Common armlines**

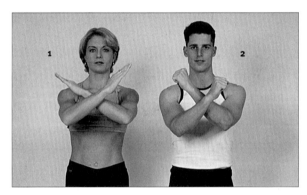

1. **Blade** 2. **Fist**

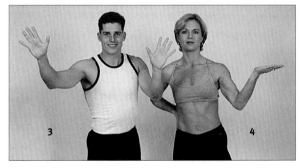

3. **Jazz (fingers spread)** 4. **Dance (palms up)**
Fig. 3.44. **Hand positions**

Cueing

Cueing is the art of informing participants of what they need to do before they do it. Successful cueing of an aerobics class results in participants doing the same thing at the same time. Let's face it, getting a group of people to do the same thing at the same time is sometimes a challenging task, not to mention that, as an instructor, you want the group to perform like this for anywhere up to one hour at a time. Aerobics participants want a challenging workout for both the body and, to a lesser extent, the mind. Participants need to feel that they have achieved success at the end of their workout and that the experience was worthwhile. As an instructor, you must learn to develop simple and effective cueing techniques so that participants will be able to follow and understand instructions.

Instructors need to be proficient in using both verbal and non-verbal cueing techniques, since effective communication skills can greatly influence an instructor's success on both an individual and class level. The successful instructor develops an affinity and rapport with participants which is measured by the response from the class.

As discussed previously in Chapter 2 (Music), before you can begin to cue effectively, you must first master your physical routine. Learn your moves first and then learn your cueing to fit the moves and music. If you forget your routine during your class, this is a good indication that you must go back and practise the physical routine.

Practice should never be underestimated. Practise your voice projection, practise naming your moves, and even your interaction skills. As a general rule, try to spend at least 30% of your preparation time on determining what you will teach; including moves, combinations, etc., and 70% on how you will teach it. This includes your cueing techniques, both verbal and non-verbal, learning curves, elements of variation, etc.

If at any time during your own teaching and learning process, you make mistakes during the routine, try not to punish yourself. All instructors make mistakes. Continue to practise to ensure optimal delivery of your class. The development of sound cueing techniques will greatly influence success for both the instructor and participant.

The cueing story

Instructors today are aware of the importance of the 'what, where, when and how' of verbal cueing. The cueing ability of experienced instructors enables them to teach highly creative patterns and choreography whilst maintaining a sense of achievement for all ability levels within their classes. The emphasis should be on the word 'teach'. Teaching takes all participants on a journey by successfully building and developing patterns and choreography.

It is important to note that, in the process of communication, participants receive 70% of information through non-verbal messages. Hence, the importance of non-verbal cueing cannot be underestimated. Signs and symbols, facial expressions, correct technique and execution of movement by the instructor, music, props and suitable exercise selection are all methods of non-verbal cueing that can be used effectively during a class.

The EZQ system (see Fig. 4.1) is a system of easily recognised, standardised visual cues that instructors can incorporate into their teaching to improve participant–instructor communication. These visual cues create a consistent format of communication in all classes. You or your centre may have your own EZQ system which your participants recognise, but the techniques for visual cueing at the next centre may be different again. It is important to standardise these techniques for cueing throughout the aerobics industry, as well as standardising names for base moves, direction and travel patterns, amongst other components of your classes.

Verbal cueing— The What, Where, When and How

The **What**, or exercise identification cue, refers to the actual move, exercise or armline that is being performed—for example, in Aerobics a grapevine, step touch, shoulder press, upright row or, for Step, a basic step, repeater or a turn step. Cues should be verbalised clearly and delivered in a consistent manner. Ensure that you are confident in your delivery by holding your head high and projecting your cues to the group.

Descriptive, footwork and rhythmic cueing will further assist participants. Descriptive cueing simply describes the movement, and will often include the footwork cues, e.g. grapevine cues would be 'step behind, step together'. Rhythmic cueing could be calling out the rhythm, such as '1 and 2', or 'run run run' for a cha-cha-cha.

The **Where**, or direction/placement cue, refers to the direction of the movement. Such cues as left, right, forward or back, side, behind will be used here. Geographical cues such as mirror, door, equipment or exit may also be used. This will make your job easier as the movement sequence increases in complexity.

The **When** or numerical/countdown cue is used to prompt participants of a change. It refers to how many repetitions remain and when to change. Instruction should commence on the fifth or sixth beat of the phrase to ensure that enough warning is provided prior to changing. As an instructor, you should learn to develop countdown cueing. On a countdown to cue the next move, your call should sound similar to the following: '4, 3, 2, next move', e.g. '4, 3, 2, grapevine'. If you attempt to count down to 1 and then cue the next move, you will find that there is inadequate time and the cues will be rushed. Remember that only a minimal amount of information will fit into that 1 or 2 beats. Keep this information clear, concise and to the point. Always cue early and be prepared.

The **How**, or quality/technique cue, refers to the way in which the movement is to be performed. The use of power words, imagery and mental stimulation can help to achieve the desired movement pattern. Such cues as big steps, long arms, high knees are all examples of the How cue. Quality/technique cues may also signal a change in intensity, pace, rhythm or offer participants correctional advice on their form or body positioning. Such cues as soft knees, wider legs, stand tall can be used here.

Additional verbal cues can be used to motivate or educate your participants during the workout. The use of intonation will help to reinforce quality cues and power words. 'It's not what you say but the way that you say it' that will get the desired response from partici-

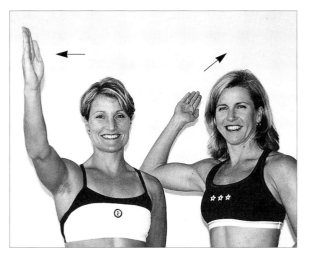
1. Backwards and forwards

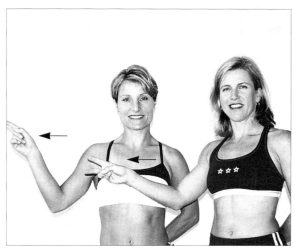
2. Side and 2's

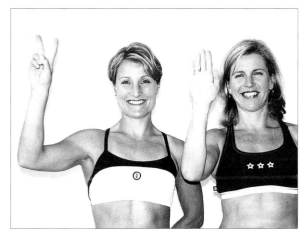
3. Countdown and hold

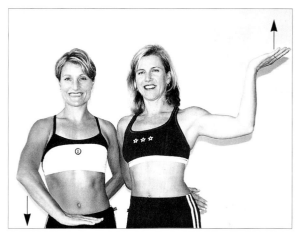
4. Low and high

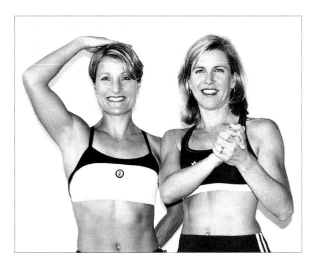
5. From the top and link combination together

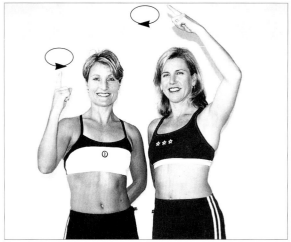
6. Circle on the spot and circle around the room

Fig. 4.1. **The EZQ system**

pants. The use of a happy or an energy charged voice and the length at which you pronounce words, e.g. 'l-o-n-g', 'squeeze', 'push' and 'pull' will attract attention and allow participants to associate the tones with the desired intensity level or technique.

General communication can be inserted throughout your class to get participants focused or to divert attention back to the instructor during the class. Such comments as 'How are you feeling?', 'You should be feeling that by now, nod if you can', 'Smile during this one' and 'The answer to the question is "yes"—are you having fun?'

To avoid overuse of your own voice or unnecessary talk in your aerobics classes, try to be aware of what to cue and when. Place your cues in a priority order, which is usually the What first, followed by the When, Where and then the How, e.g. 'Step touch right, after 4, 3, 2, go, bigger steps'.

> **ᛟ ᛟ Drill ᛟ ᛟ**
>
> Footwork cueing, directional cueing, rhythmic cueing, numerical cueing, visual cueing and travel cues will all fit into the What, Where, When and How techniques of cueing. Develop a simple combination and identify each one of these cues and practise in front of a mirror and with a partner.

As an instructor, aim to practise the What, Where, When cues first. When you are confident with these, aim to include the How (quality and technique), praise, interaction and your non-verbal communication techniques. Remember to cue in advance to provide adequate warning.

Non-verbal cueing

Non-verbal cueing can be classified into six different type of cues, and each of these can assist in the What, Where, When and How.

1. Signs or symbols

Signs or symbols may represent direction, intensity, number of repetitions and moves/patterns. These cues can either be initiated by the instructor or can be from an extrinsic source. The EZQ system (see Fig. 4.1) has a set of universally used cues that are easy to recognise and follow for instructors and participants alike. Signs or symbol cues can either be hand signals, clapping, circuit cards or thumbs up, signalling correct exercise execution.

2. Facial expressions

Facial expressions are a large part of an instructor's style. Eye contact can be used to acknowledge progress or effort, to single out individuals or good performances, to show direction, and pre-empt other cues. A smile, eye contact, nod of the head or other gesture will help to encourage participants. Participants need to know that they are not only being supervised, but that they are exercising correctly. The use of facial expressions will help participants to feel at ease and get to learn your personality too. Meet and greet participants with your eyes and smile regularly before, during and after your classes. A smile will always attract another smile. Be genuine and sincere with your facial expressions.

3. Music

Music assists the cueing process as it contains in-built cues that are in rhythm, phrasing and lyric composition.

4. Exercise selection and progress

Exercise selection and progress. Simple and logical changes are crucial to ensure effective cueing. Select your exercises to allow for easy transition from one move to the next. When designing travel or direction changes, shapes or geographical cues within the room can assist you with non-verbal cueing.

5. Body language

Body language is an important part of communication. The position of our bodies can often display our comfort or distress with various situations. When instructing, use correct body alignment and appropriate body positioning to demonstrate new or existing moves. As an instructor, don't be afraid to turn your body side-on to the group in order to show another angle when demonstrating. Move around your group and stand alongside participants to allow them to copy your body positioning. If you do need to touch your participants to correct their technique, always touch hard parts of their body such as shoulders or elbows, never touch soft points such as bottoms or stomachs.

6. Visual previewing

Visual previewing is a great technique to employ when instructing, provided it is used well. Visual previews involve placing participants into a holding pattern and asking the class to watch while you perform the next move, or when you add an element of variation to the current move. The emphasis must be placed on the word 'move'. Visual previewing of one or two moves is acceptable. Visual previewing is used incorrectly when the instructor tries to preview a new 32-count combination without breaking down the choreography. Don't use visual previews if your moves are so complicated that you are unable to teach them by layering small changes at a time. Ensure that you get your participants to the final product by taking them on a journey through the teaching and learning experience. This will allow for maximum retention of the move and ensure that all participants will confidently learn the move you are teaching.

If you use the visual preview throughout your class, be careful your participants' intensity level does not drop. If you continually place your group into a holding pattern whilst you demonstrate the next sequence of moves, the intensity of the workout can decrease dramatically. Remember, you are there to teach, not to demonstrate, so always use visual previewing correctly.

Elements of effective cueing

Consistency

It is one thing to know in theory how to cue effectively, it is another to be able to show consistency with these skills year in, year out, or even from one class to the next. Consistency comes with practice. Practice allows you to develop a bank of easy-to-follow, easily understood cues. Learn to use the cues regularly and vary them to suit the situation.

Keep it direct and to the point

To ensure that cueing is easy to follow for all participant levels, make sure your cueing is direct and to the point. Ensure that your cues are not verbose, otherwise you may be rushing to get the message across. Participants must be able to react to instructions quickly and with confidence for the class to be successful and to maintain a certain flow. Remember, when to cue is as equally as important as what to cue.

Well timed

Use music phrasing to 'time' your cues. Work with the music, not over it, when delivering cues. Always make your way around the room when instructing, to check such factors as music volume throughout the room, and the level of microphone sound. These factors will determine if your participants can hear your cues or not. If you are not sure of your voice volume, ask your participants at regular intervals whether they can hear you well. Ask for a simple response such as a head nod or thumbs up for yes, or vice versa for no.

Visibility

When instructing, always be visible to all participants. Where you stand and how you position yourself (whether you are facing the class, the mirror, or facing away from the class) can dramatically effect the impact of your cues. Change your position regularly and don't be afraid to leave the stage or instructing area to work around your class. Always check first that you can see your participants. If you can't see them, the participants can certainly not see you. Make adjustments throughout the class to ensure you have optimal visual impact on your group.

Exercise selection

At the initial planning stage of your classes, you must firstly select the appropriate exercises or moves to be used in your choreography. The progression from one exercise to another is a crucial element in effective cueing. When planning choreography or your class structure, aim to make changes logical and simple. Avoid making too many changes at once, as too much information will result in verbose and rushed cueing. In addition to this, avoid long sequences of complex skills. Try to mix the more complex choreography with simple moving to allow participants to focus on working their body and not just their mind. Not only will this keep the intensity high throughout the class, but it will allow you, the instructor, to have 'time out' from continuous cueing.

Keep it simple

Simplicity will always be the key to effective cueing and teaching. The KISS (Keep It So Simple) method will assist you in your delivery. Try not to get carried away with excessive cueing, or planning too many combinations in your classes. The more experience you gain as an aerobics instructor, the easier it will be for you to know what needs to be said and demonstrated and what doesn't.

Voice projection

Instructing with a microphone has made teaching a much easier process on the voice. At all times, with or without a microphone, consider not only your projection but your tone and pitch. Focus on your breathing and comfort level when cueing. Make frequent adjustments to the mouthpiece on the microphone if it is picking up your breathing or if it shifts during class. Avoid unnecessary talk in your classes; occasional silence is okay.

Adjustments

When you can see one participant or many participants performing exercises incorrectly, try to remedy this immediately. For reasons of safety and exercise effectiveness, don't ever let incorrect technique be ignored in your class. Adjustments in your classes can be made to the group as a whole, to a subset of the group or to one person amongst a group by using eye contact and other body cues. Avoid obviously singling out one individual within the group. Move towards the participant and turn off your microphone so you can make the necessary adjustments one on one.

Other techniques could include a more hands-on approach of moving towards a single participant and making gestures towards the particular body part that needs adjustment. It is advisable to ask permission before touching a participant. A simple 'May I adjust your technique?' will elicit a yes or no response either verbally or non-verbally. Avoid touching 'soft' body parts such as the stomach or gluteals. If touching is not appropriate, stand alongside that participant so they can imitate your movement pattern, or touch the target body part on your own body. Use key words to give participants a better idea of how to correctly execute the move. Always follow a correction with praise.

Balance your teaching process

Two methods are mostly used for balancing your teaching processes during classes. These are:

Automatic

Focus on one or two types of cues, depending on the class component, e.g. in an aerobic conditioning phase, you may wish to focus on direction and action words to recall moves or to increase intensity. These cues may be used for each class component.

Self-awareness technique

Identify how you normally cue. Try to develop styles of cueing that you may rarely use. Join other instructors' classes and pay particular attention to their cueing techniques, and compare these to your own. Try new voice tones and motivational sayings to add variety to your teaching methods, and spend additional time planning a more creative class format or style. Read motivational books or the latest research for new tips, pointers and educational pieces for your group.

Successful cueing involves the identification of some simple teaching techniques. As an instructor, each component of cueing must be understood and utilised during classes for it to be effective. Not only the what, when, where and how cues, but your EZQ signs, music phrasing, body language, facial expression, visual preview and imagery. To be a great instructor, continue to practise all elements of cueing, and tackle each class with motivation and preparation. All methods of cueing are equally important to enhance your teaching technique and to assist you in adding the element of variation. Remember, when to cue is equally as important as what to cue.

Teaching Methodologies

Enjoyment, achievement and fun would certainly be amongst the goals for participants in an aerobics class, and using a range of teaching methods is a great way to achieve these aims. Traditionally, aerobics classes were performed on the spot and with very little travel. Organised action put a stop to this stationary form of aerobics by introducing different formations such as lines and 'organising' a range of simple-to-follow activities. Other teaching techniques can be used to sequence moves and develop combinations. Techniques range from a simple 'follow me' style of teaching through to more structured teaching methods.

Regardless of which type of class you are instructing, organised action and additional approaches to teaching will show you that even the simplest technique can allow creativity and optimise the potential for all movement patterns. The simplistic nature of organised action and the more challenging advanced teaching methods can ensure success when implemented and used correctly in your classes.

Choreography in aerobics classes refers to the art of planning and arranging movements to music. Easy-to-follow choreography has gained immense popularity over the years. Many instructors will lack confidence in preparing and presenting choreography; but the application of teaching methods will enable them to prepare successful choreography. A teaching method is a technique used to develop choreography. A learning curve describes the stages or progression of learning that takes place. Because of the emphasis on teaching and learning, participants are able to master the movement sequences and thereby make the workout much more enjoyable and effective for them.

Teaching methods will enable you to teach in some progressive order so that you can use your base moves over and over again, but the journey to the finished product will always be different. The learning curve is how you get there or build up a block of choreography; the teaching method is the technique, e.g. the use of link or add-on. The learning progressions are like road signs in the way that they give you directions on how to teach. In order for an individual to really learn, three stages of learning must be completed. These are the cognitive, psycho-motor and affective domains of learning, which include seeing, doing and feeling. This chapter covers all aspects of both teaching and learning.

1. Linear progression

This is the simplest way of teaching freestyle choreography where a combination or routine is not developed. Linear progression involves making one small change at a time when sequencing moves together. This change will either be an armline, a leg pattern or base move, or by adding an element of variation. Linear progression can be classified as a 'topless' workout because, unlike combinations, you do not need to continually go 'from the top' or back to Move A. You can repeat a move, but it does not have to be in any particular pattern.

Zig-zag is a variation of linear progression. It involves making a number of changes, then reversing the sequence up the ladder, back down the ladder and then progressing with more moves.

Practical application — Zig-zag

Counts	Move	Lower Body	Travel	Direction	Upper Body
1–32	A	16 x step touch	OTS	Face front	No armline
1–32	A	16 x step touch	OTS	Face front	Bicep curls*
1–32	B	8 x dbl step touch*	OTS	Face front	Bicep curl
1–32	B	8 x dbl step touch	OTS	Face front	Upright row*
1–32	C	8 x grapevines*	OTS	Face front	Upright row
1–32	C	8 x grapevines	OTS	Face front	Low row*
1–32	D	4 x grapevine with 3 alt. leg curls*	OTS	Face front	Low row
1–32	D	4 x grapevine with 3 alt. leg curls	OTS	Face front	Reverse curl*

Now zig-zag back from the grapevine with 3 alt. curls back up to the first move.

* indicates the changing factor.

Considerations for linear progression

Effective transitions. In linear progression, plan each transition thoroughly. An effective transition refers to the ease at which moves can be changed from the previous move to the next. Cue in advance and know where you are going for the next move. Balance all aspects of movement patterns and planes of the body.

Moves utilised. Variety will be the key when selecting your base moves. To get the most from your base moves, use the elements of variation. This will make your movement selection and possibilities endless and creative. Attempt to have an even balance of non-impact, low impact and high impact base moves (but not in the warm-up). When adding variations to your high impact base moves, remember to do no more than 32 consecutive repetitions per foot strike pattern and do no more than 8 hops on one leg or 4 repeater lift moves. This will ensure that a balance between high and low impact moves applies for all ability and fitness levels within your group.

Direction and travel. When adding travel, combine forward, backward, lateral, rotational and on-the-spot variations. These will vary the repetitive frictional and impact forces of continually working on the spot.

2. Pyramid method

Just like the shape of a pyramid, the repetitions of a move or sequence are either gradually increased or decreased. Repetitions are gradually increased to fit both the musical phrase and the ease of progression. This is used to build repeater moves. Reverse pyramid refers to the reduction of repetitions, which leads to an increase in the complexity of the combination. The main advantage of the pyramid technique is that, like linear progression, participants can focus on form, technique, intensity and committing to the move.

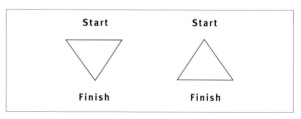

Fig. 5.1. **Reverse pyramid and pyramid**

Practical application

Counts	Move	Lower Body	Travel	Direction
1–16	A	8 x alt. touch step side R,L	OTS	Face front
17–32	B	4 x alt. double touch step side (RR, LL x 4)	OTS	Face front
1–32	C	4 x alt. four touch steps side (RRRR, LLLL x 4))	OTS	Face front

Reduce repetitions to 4, 2, 2 then 2, 1, 1 reps.

Counts	Move	Lower Body	Travel	Direction
1–32	A	16 x squats narrow	OTS	Face front
1–32	B	16 x squats wide	OTS	Face front

Reduce repetitions to 8 of each move, then 4, 2 and possibly 1 rep. of each move (depending on complexity).

3. Add-on method

This is also referred to as the memory or building block method. In the add-on method only one move is added at a time. That is, A, A+B, A+B+C, A+B+C+D. With this method, Move A is always the starting point and no matter what move sequence you are up to, you must always go back to Move A to restart or to go 'from the top'. It is important to note that the Add-on method can also be done in blocks of choreography, e.g. Block A + Block B.

Add-on is a simple process for teaching and learning. The problem that may occur with this method is when we add too many moves together and it is difficult to recall the sequence. A maximum number of 4–8 moves is recommended.

Practical application

Counts	Move	Lower body	Travel	Direction
Teach A				
1–8	A	1 x dbl grapevine	Lat	Face front
Teach B				
1–8	B	4 x step curl	OTS	Face front
Join A + B leading right then left.				
Teach C				
1–8	C	2 x ezy walk	OTS	Face front
Join A + B + C + C leading right then left. (Move C is repeated so that a 32-count block is completed.)				
Teach D				
1–8	D	4 x alt. knee lift	OTS	Face front
Join A + B + C + D leading right then left.				

4. Link method

Commonly described as 'part to whole' teaching, the link method involves Moves A and B being taught and then linked together, and then the same is done for Moves C and D. Finally, Moves (A+B) are joined to Moves (C+D) to develop a four-move combination. Further linking can take place (E + F) and (G + I) to develop a large combination.

Practical application

Counts	Move	Lower Body	Travel	Direction
Teach A				
1–16	A	4 x grapevine R, L	Lat	Face front
Teach B				
17–32	B	4 x ezy walk R	OTS	Face front
Join (A + B).				
Teach C				
1–16	C	8 x heels fwd	OTS	Face front
Teach D				
17–32	D	8 x squat (feet together)		Face front
Join (C + D).				
Finally, join (A + B) and (C + D).				
The option exists to reduce the reps as follows:				
1–8	A	2 x grapevine R, L	Lat	Face front
7–16	B	2 x ezy walk R	OTS	Face front
17–24	C	4 x heels fwd, R, L, R, L	OTS	Face front
25–32	D	4 x squat (feet together)	OTS	Face front

Repeat the combination, and then repeat combination using opposite footwork (right/left balance).

5. Holding patterns addition

Holding patterns can be used throughout your classes when you need to give either yourself or your participants a mind break or before teaching a new block of choreography. The holding pattern addition technique allows you to buy time and gives your participants time to catch up with the moves. A holding pattern can be inserted between moves as you teach them or to expand the original length of your routine. Your original number of moves are taught in a sequence and then a holding pattern/move is placed between these sub-components. When teaching moves, the holding move will be inserted as follows: Move A + (holding move) + Move B + (holding move) + Move C + (holding move) + Move D + (holding move). It can also be used in between (A + B) + (holding move) + (C+D) + (holding move).

Practical application

Counts	Move	Lower Body	Travel	Direction
Teach A				
1–16	A	8 x step touch R, L	OTS	Face front
Teach B				
1–16	B	4 x grapevines R, L	Lat	Face front
= 32 counts (1 block)				
Then introduce the holding pattern: walk fwd 1, 2, 3, jump; repeat bwd				
1–16	A	8 x step touch R,L	OTS	Face front
1–16	H/m*	2 x walk fwd/bwd	Fwd/bwd	Face front
1–16	B	4 x alt. grapevines R, L	Lat	Face front
1–16	H/m*	4 x walk fwd/bwd	Fwd/bwd	Face front
=64 counts (2 blocks)				
*H/m = holding move				

To increase the intensity, turn the walk into a jog or double jog. This teaching method can also be useful in both muscle conditioning or Step classes.

6. Add and subtract

Following along the lines of the add-on method, the add and subtract method adds one component at a time. However, instead of continuously adding on new moves, as one new move is added, one of the established moves is subtracted. This is also known as 'Top 'n Tail'.

Practical application

(A + B)(A + B)(A + B) + C
(B + C)(B + C)(B + C) + D
(C + D)(C + D)(C + D) + E, etc.

7. Layering

When a combination or pattern of moves has been learnt and established, your participants should be able to repeat these without too much cueing from you. This is a good time to make gradual changes to the pattern by using the layering technique. Layering refers to making simple changes, one at a time, to obtain more mileage from the original combination. This technique allows for a logical, easy transition from a simple to a complex routine. As a result of these gradual changes, exercise intensity is not compromised. Layering is achieved by adding elements of variation.

Practical application

Counts	Move	Lower Body	Travel	Direction
1–8	A	4 x step touches R,L,R,L	OTS	Face front
9–16	B	4 x touch step (side) R,L,R,L	OTS	Face front
17–24	C	4 x jumping jacks	OTS	Face front
25–32	D	8 x jog	OTS	Face front
Now try to layer the following changes one at a time:				
1.		A = travel fwd and becomes a step jump		
2.		B = 2 x dbl touch step R, L		
3.		C = 2 x squat jack		
4.		D = travel bwd		

Remember, the layers should be gradual and must be made one at a time. After layering Move A, go back and repeat the combination several times over. When you feel the participants are confident with the change, then add the next layer. Again, go back and repeat the new combination, and so on until the new sequence has been learnt. Other changes that can be layered include rhythm, direction, shapes, armlines and even noises or sound effects.

Variations of this technique can include splitting the class. Half of the group may lead with the left leg and the other half of the group with the right leg to complete this combination. In this case, each half of the group will be performing the combination moving away from each other. They can then change sides or turn to face the back. At the same time the instructor also changes position to be placed in front of the group at the back of the room (the group is facing the back of the room) and both groups perform the combination on their opposite lead leg.

8. Organised action

Organised action is a not a new concept. Sporting teams and coaches have employed organised action drills and techniques into their training sessions for years. These techniques add the elements of variety, skill development, team interaction and cohesion to any session. By making the most of the patterns utilised, intensity will be high, interest levels will be high and the effectiveness of the workout will be high. The interaction between your group or team will create a positive social atmosphere and allow you to demonstrate to your group your creative flair, planning and preparation ability.

The obvious advantages of utilising organised action in your classes are listed below, along with planning considerations and practical applications.

Advantages

Grouping
Try to group your participants to allow for maximum social interaction and successful performances. The various formations you select will either enhance or detract from these considerations.

Variety
With your regular participants there will be a tendency for them to hold or reserve their favourite spot in the room for every class. By selecting new travel patterns with your group, you will move participants from their comfort zones and create interest with new formats.

Value
As an instructor you will be able to gain maximum value and mileage from your base moves by varying your travel patterns and class formats. As only a small number of base moves will be used at one time, their repetition will add the elements of variety and fun.

Change in instructor focus
Rather than focussing on choreography, your emphasis can shift to organising activities and motivating your participants. It takes the instructor away from the front and places him/her at the centre of the activities. This allows the instructor to become involved in the socialisation occurring within the class.

Consideration must be given to the physical, mental and social aspects of health with planning your classes. The body or physical aspects can be challenged throughout your class. Choreography allows the mental aspect of health to be covered, as well as having the participants feel good about themselves and their workout. The social aspects of health can be catered for with organised action. A friendly and motivating atmosphere is developed within this phase of the class. This can certainly be used to the advantage of the instructor, with participants feeling fun, enjoyment and satisfaction from this phase of the workout.

Planning considerations

Do not attempt to use organised action in your class without thorough planning and consideration of the following factors:
- the size and shape of the room;
- presence or absence of pillars, poles or equipment in the room;
- use of microphone and location of the sound system;
- the number of people likely to attend;
- the ability level of your participants;
- allowing for pre-class setting-up if needed;
- remembering the aims of the workout and your role in successfully implementing organised action;
- the movement combinations selected to ensure that your participants can follow and feel good about the success of the activity and their role in that success;
- using a log book summary to effectively and efficiently plan your moves (see Appendix II);
- developing an organisational plan and diagram that will allow you to scan your set-up when necessary.

Practical application

Perimeter groups

Effective class organisation

Have your group form a large circle around the room from either a power walk or jogging activity. This circle formation should be attempted before you group the class and divide them. Use the walls as landmarks, e.g. 'Go to your nearest wall and face the centre'. Attempt to make each of the four groups/clusters as even as possible. Each of the groups A to D will have a different base move. Before the command of change, each group will be instructed to look at the next move being performed by the group on their right. This will be their next move as they prepare to travel to the next station around the room. On the command of change, each group will move to their right and change.

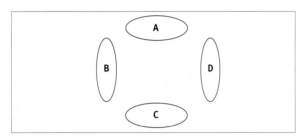

Fig. 5.2. **Cluster circuit**

Variations

More than four groups can be made. After all of the groups have been to every station and they have performed each of the moves, the same formation can remain and each group can be given a completely new move. The centre of the room can be used as another variation and the groups can come back together in the middle facing the front and perform each move added together, i.e. A + B + C + D. This can be repeated several times. The participants can then be instructed to go back into their groups and then new moves can be given.

Effective class organisation

Organise participants in lines against all four walls. All groups will be instructed to perform the same base move or holding pattern. On command, line A will power-walk/jog/sprint across the room and back. Once they have returned to their original place, line B will go, followed by C and then D. All groups will then rotate to the right and a new base move or holding pattern will be established. Repeat the circuit until each group has been positioned at each side of the room. Ensure that your groups are instructed not to turn too fast or race each other to the other side. It is potentially dangerous to touch the floor or wall before turning.

If numbers are insufficient for four lines, organise two lines at opposite walls. In this formation the lines face each other and can either move to the centre and back or they can cross over completely. For larger classes make two or more sets of facing lines. This can also be combined with partner work. Partners can either be side by side or directly opposite each other on the other side of the room. You must instruct the partners to always cross by their right shoulders or their left shoulders. Holding moves must be established early and regularly changed.

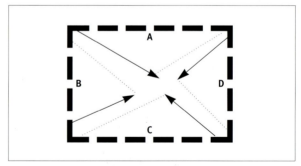

Fig. 5.4. **Four-sided triangle circuit**

Effective class organisation

Line your participants in their groups along each wall and give them a base move or holding pattern to perform. The right side is the start of the line. In a small class, one person in each group (at the start of the line)

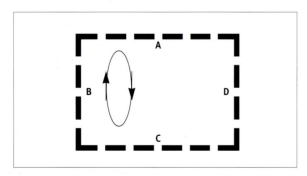

Fig. 5.3. **Four-sided circuit with sprint**

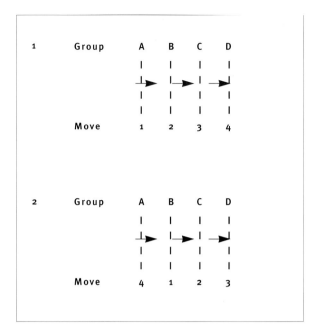

Fig. 5.5. **Non-rotating circuits**

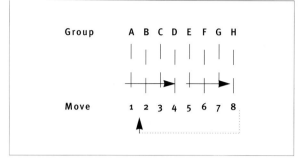

Fig. 5.6. **Rotating line circuit**

will travel to the centre. In a large group, increase this to three to four people. When the participants reach the centre they will perform an exercise there before returning to the opposite end of the line.

Variations

The base move can be travelled to move in to the centre, e.g. flick kick. Participants would then jog or power walk to the end of the line. Participants could slide or side step into the centre and out again without having to perform the exercise in the centre. This would increase the pace of the circuit. Groups A to D each have their own move and once each person has travelled in to the centre, all groups could rotate to the right.

Line circuits

Effective class organisation

Give each group a base move before organisation starts. Instruct group to move into a smaller space to make group formations easier to organise. Select the four closest participants to you, or four regular participants, to be the line leaders and form four straight lines (see Fig. 5.5). (This circuit can be done with four to eight lines.)

Give each group a different move. Instruct groups to look to their right to see their next move, i.e. non-rotating. On the command of change each group will stay where they are and perform their new move. As it will be difficult for group D to see the next move from line A, you must stay with group D and give them their next move.

Variations

Lines can power-walk or jog to their right, left or fwd/bwd, depending on your command, before changing moves. After all four moves have been completed by each group, the moves can be joined together into a combination and performed to the front. These four base moves can have travel added where applicable.

Effective class organisation

The set up will be similar to the four line circuit and each line will need to look to their right for the next move. On the command of change, each line will physically move to the line on their right and resume the next move. Line H will be led by you to the other end of the circuit and shown the first move. (This circuit can be done with four to eight lines — see Fig. 5.6.)

Variation

The eight moves can be joined together, travel patterns added and performed to the front. Group H can travel 1½ laps around the room before starting the first move. All lines can jog/walk to their right or left (see cast-offs) before changing to their next line. The front position of each group can continually change. Have all groups face the front, then on the next change have all groups face the right, and then on the next change, the back, etc. You will always need to take group H on to the first position and give them their next move to avoid confusion.

Relays

Effective class organisation

Have the class perform a holding pattern/move, e.g. walk or jog OTS while you organise them into four lines. Ensure that the participants are close together in their

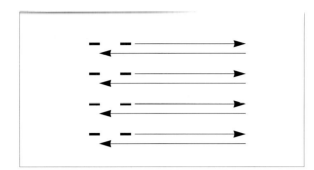

Fig. 5.7. **Single-end relays**

lines. The first person in each group jogs/walks to the other end of the room and back again. On their return, they tag the next person to start and they go to the back of the line.

You will need to continually change the move your group is performing. Ensure that you instruct your participants on the dangers of travelling or turning too quickly. Motivate your participants to maintain a good pace so that all groups can start and finish together. Avoid strong competition, as this can motivate some participants and turn off others. Instruct all participants not to touch the wall or floor before turning.

Variations

Upon reaching the far end, the relay runner can perform an exercise that you call out or demonstrate. Another alternative is a circuit card listing four alternative exercises, e.g. 1) 8 x knee lift, 2) 8 x star jumps, 3) 8 x astride jumps, 4) 8 x flick kicks. The circuit will then be repeated four times so that each of the four exercises can be performed each new time. Novelty exercises may be thrown in, e.g. 8 x frog hops.

Have a halfway station so that an exercise is performed halfway down and then another at the end.

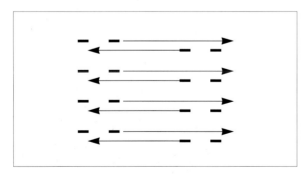

Fig. 5.8. **Double-ended relays**

Props may be carried or collected from end to end such as oranges, balloons, beanbags or hats. Relays always work well for theme classes. These could include partner classes, Christmas, Easter, country and western or Halloween.

Effective class organisation

Have the class perform a holding move, e.g. walk or jog OTS, and set up four straight lines down the room. Cut each line evenly in half and send each half to the opposite ends of the room. The lines must face the centre of the room, facing each other. Give clear explanations of what is expected of each group. The first person in each group on one side of the room jogs/walks across to their facing team, tags the first person and moves to the end of the new line. The tagged runner then repeats this sequence to the opposite end of the room. All runners must return to their original starting position for one circuit to be completed.

Once the action is re-established, the instructor takes the group through a range of moves. You must position yourself in a place where all of your participants can see you, yet you are not interfering with any runners. Power walking may be the most appropriate intensity level to aim for, as relay runners may take the intensity too high.

Variations

Set up a halfway station in line with yourself and have the runner perform the desired number of exercises before they move on to tag the next runner. Another variation is to set each runner up with a partner. The pair must run and, where applicable, perform a partner move together.

Cast-offs

Effective class organisation

While the group is walking or running OTS, divide them into four even lines. Instruct each group that they will be following their leader by walking to the front of the line, turning to their right or left, depending on your command, walking to the back of the room or far end and then returning to their original position. Keep varying the holding move and the direction in which the leader must take their group. The element of surprise will add enjoyment to this exercise. Instruct every participant to make their way right to the front

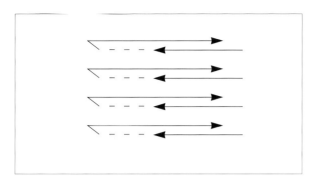

Fig. 5.9. **Cast-offs**

and then right to the back before turning. Try to keep the pace similar by instructing either a power walk or a jog.

Variation

Organise your groups and formation by requesting those who may wish to jog in the next exercise to move to the left side of the room, and those wishing to power walk to move to the right side of the room. It will then be easy to divide groups by fitness levels by having a jogging half of the room and a power-walking half of the room.

The two outside groups can walk down between the two inside groups. This is followed by the two inside groups walking out and around the outside groups. Continual cast offs can be performed. Don't break up the walks with a holding move. As soon as the groups return from their walk to the right, send them immediately to the left.

Shapes

1. Basic circle
Effective class organisation

Participants walk/jog in a circle. Ensure that you change the direction regularly. Avoid just calling out a change at random as half of the class may turn and the other half may not. This may also cause collisions within the group. Some alternative ways to instruct the change in direction can include:

- Count down before a change to prepare your group, e.g. 'Ready to change after 4, 3, 2, change direction'. A clap can accompany the cue change direction to attract additional attention.
- While the group is travelling, warn them they are going to stop. Perform a holding move on the spot and then signal their direction change. You may even keep them moving in the same direction and not change the direction until after the next holding move.
- From the start of the new move, instruct the class that they will be taking a set number of steps in each direction. Again, count them down before the change so that each participant will change simultaneously.

Variations

You can also join the circle and become the leader. Peel the line off diagonally across the room and continue in the opposite direction. Another variation is termed 'in and out', where you simply move towards the centre of the circle and out. Like the Pied Piper, you can change armlines and leg patterns with this leader set-up. Ensure that both verbal and non-verbal cues are used.

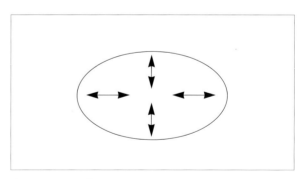

Fig. 5.11. **In and out**

2. Double circle
Effective class organisation

Have two complete circles travelling in opposite directions, or one circle can be performing a stationary move while the other travels. The stationary move can be alternated between groups.

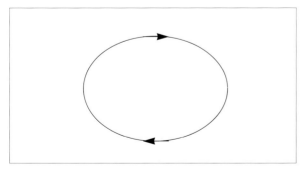

Fig. 5.10. **Basic circle**

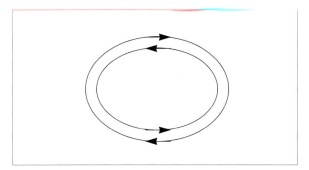

Fig. 5.12. **Double circle**

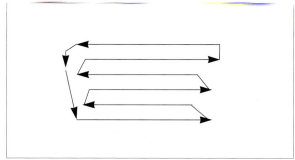

Fig. 5.14. **Snakes**

3. The Spiral
Effective class organisation

You will join the line and instruct each participant to be no more than 1 metre apart from the person in front of them. Lead the group slightly inwards and keep circling closer and closer to the centre, as in a spiral. Just as you are about to reach the centre, command a change in direction and the spiral will unwind. The last participant now becomes the leader and they must be instructed to widen the circle. Eventually the original circle formation will develop. In addition to this, instead of the whole group changing direction together, you as the leader can turn around and lead the group back out of the spiral. This becomes more complex, but is an exciting alternative as you spiral in both directions.

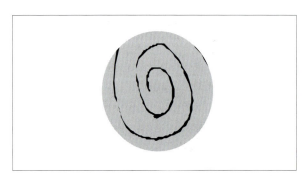

Fig. 5.13. **The spiral**

Snakes
Effective class organisation

You will join the line and instruct each participant to be no more than 1 metre apart from the person in front of them. Lead the group out of the circle formation and down along the walls of the room. Cast off to the left and have each participant stay close to the person in front of them. The snake can be taken across the room and back again. A simple power walk or jog can be performed throughout the snake, or moves can vary. Instruct your class to make move changes only at the end of the line. The snake can also lead the group into a circle formation.

Novelty and themes

When participants reach the centre of the room, have them call out a particular sound, sound effect or cheer as they reach the closest point. An alternative can be a novelty move, e.g. 'Jump on your surfboard', 'Ski down the slopes'. Each participant pretends to perform this action and then, on command, returns to the outside of the circle.

Numbering

Give each participant a number from 1 to 4 (more or less, depending on group size). While each participant performs a holding move, the instructor calls out a number and everyone with that number then advances to the centre of the room and back again. An alternative to this can be that each number, ie. 1 to 4, also represents a move. On the call of '1', the participants make their way to the centre of the room and then start to perform their move. The entire class then continues to perform this move while the participants make their way back to the outside of the room. On the command of '4', the participants numbered 4 move to the centre and then start performing their move. The entire class then joins in with this new move until this sequence is repeated for all numbers.

Considerations for organised action

1. **Music volume.** When setting up your organised action formation, the volume of the music should be decreased slightly so that all your participants can hear the instructions. Each direction change or group organisation needs to be heard and understood immediately, particularly if each group is performing a different activity.

2. **Intensity levels.** If an activity takes you too long to set up or organise, then you should seriously consider whether it should be included in your class. If your participants have to be kept in a holding pattern for too long or you take too long explaining the set up, the intensity level of each participant will drop dramatically. Attempt smooth transitions and effective use of class time.

3. **Cueing.** Your verbal cues and instructions should be clear, concise and easy to follow. Gestures can be used to accompany and enhance your verbal commands. The EZQ system can be incorporated to ensure that your cues are recognisable and visible at all times. Your verbal commands will ensure that you stay in control throughout the activities. If your planning fails, e.g. the leaders mistake their left from their right in a cast-off or chaos erupts, remain calm. Holding patterns will be useful to reorganise your groups and start all over again.

4. **Positioning.** You need to be visible to all participants at all times during the activities. When planning your organisation, consider both the shape of the room and the selected activity, in order to decide on the position that will provide good visibility for all participants. This will maximise class control and contact with your group. Stay close and in control of the entire group throughout the activity and avoid getting lost in the crowd. Avoid getting stuck in the middle of the group formation by continually changing your position and having to weave your way out through the groups. This can cause collisions, interruptions and may effect intensity levels or group momentum.

5. **Back to basics.** Any form of choreography or complex move sequences will add confusion during group changeovers. Have your own memory bank of moves planned for organised action so that they can easily be expanded through simple and interesting variations. The organised action phase needs to be a part of the whole class, not a separate entity. Ensure that the activities flow along with the total picture of the class and keep your participants moving.

6. **Preparation time.** The time you put into preparing your class and specific activities will pay off. A prepared instructor is a successful instructor. Planning does not just include one set of activities. It may include many activities that can be used as Plan B when all else fails. If things do go wrong, it is your responsibility to correct them. Your preparation time will effect your delivery and outcomes.

✂ ✂ Action Plan ✂ ✂

Plan thoroughly, consider all formations to suit your room size and the size of the group.

✂ Stay visible and in control through effective positioning.

✂ Monitor noise and instructional volume.

✂ Basic is best, with a lot of repetition and motivation.

✂ Practice will make perfect each and every time.

✂ Be the teacher and stay in control of each activity and each group.

✂ Establish an action plan (or Plan B) for times of need

9. Pre-choreography

Pre-choreographed classes were the first ever offered to aerobics participants and they have been the foundation of aerobics ever since. The freestyle form of aerobics has since evolved from instructor creativity and an overall improvement in teaching skills. Pre-choreographed classes come in all forms from Hi-Lo classes to muscle-conditioning workouts. Pre-choreography involves the same format or routines being followed for a set number of weeks or months at a time. The introduction of 'Body Pump' by Les Mills© has contributed to a renewed interest in pre-choreography, and this structured barbell class is becoming increasingly popular in many countries throughout the world.

Pre-choreography applies quality control strategies as used by leading businesses in all industries. Like chain hamburger outlets, the pre-choreographed class can offer participants the opportunity to consume the same workout at any number of fitness centres in local cities, states, provinces or countries. In pre-choreographed classes participants can learn routines to enhance their success. The programs are athletic and simple in nature, with a strong focus on getting results geared to the mass market.

The pre-choreographed class such as a barbell or Hi-Lo class has numerous advantages:

- Intensity levels remain consistent. Depending on the target audience, the class will reliably deliver the appropriate intensity level.
- Because the choreography stays the same for several months, participants can gauge their own improvements week by week and enjoy the feeling of achievement once they have mastered the routines, whereas in regular choreographed aerobics they may not have the opportunity to try the routine again.
- The consistency of the workout means that participants work within their comfort zones at all times.
- The instructor can be more relaxed and focus on teaching, educating and motivating participants rather than continually trying to remember or create new choreography.
- Classes are not dependent on one instructor, as many instructors can teach the same class. Hence, if a key instructor leaves your centre, the pre-choreographed program will not be affected.
- Aerobics co-ordinators can monitor the program standards more closely, as the product will consistently be of a high standard.
- Less preparation time is required of the instructor. This is ideal for instructors who only work part-time in the industry.
- Pre-choreography is an ideal way to introduce newcomers to the aerobics floor.
- Different types of classes establish and maintain a focus on a specific target market.
- This program can account for an increase in fitness centre income due to the fact that newcomers, advanced, older or younger participants of both sexes can all exercise comfortably in the same environment.
- Pre-choreography explodes the myths of the aerobics floor, i.e. that aerobics is only for women and the dance-orientated.
- Pre-choreographed classes can be very complex or very basic, depending on the target group.

Application of teaching methods

When applying the teaching methods to your classes there are a number of considerations that must be made. These include:

Using a range of teaching methods

As you try out the drills and activities to understand and utilise the teaching methods, you will notice that not just one, but a number of learning curves, can be applied to develop the final product, as follows:

add-on ➔ reverse pyramid ➔ layer or
reverse pyramid ➔ link ➔ holding pattern addition

Each phase of the workout can also be accompanied by teaching methods. Teaching methods can be used in the warm-up, cardiovascular, muscle-conditioning and cool-down phases of your classes.

The teaching methods will become an essential part of each and every one of your classes. Take your participants on a journey through the learning process with your selected teaching methods. Each participant will learn in different ways and at different speeds, but they will benefit so much more from the time you spend developing your combinations. When you do arrive at the finished product, it will be easier for participants to perform the moves and the variations of these moves because of the fact that they have actually learnt the moves along the way with you.

Variations of all teaching methods exist, so that you can experiment and get the most out of each method.

Practice will make each teaching method easier to use. Soon you will be using them without even realising it.

Beginner vs advanced

Certain teaching methods can be classified as either beginner or advanced methods. A simple method for beginners may be linear progression. It is easy to follow and only one change is made at a time. More advanced methods for participants are the add-on and link methods, which involve many moves to create combinations and require a good memory. You must learn to evaluate the fitness and ability level of your group and apply the appropriate teaching methods.

Make it a goal to master each of the teaching methods, both in theory and practice. The application of each method can help make your classes fun, interesting and varied. A great instructor will ensure that his/her participants learn their routines well, and feel as though they have really achieved in the classes conducted by this motivated—and motivating—teacher.

Drill

Find another instructor as a partner, and develop a four-move combination.

Partner 1 teaches the four moves, using the add-on method.

Partner 2 teaches the four moves, using the link method.

Use the same four base moves and select another teaching method each, and develop the learning curve.

You may decide that one teaching method was more suitable than another, which often depends on the actual combination. A different combination may be best taught using another method, which is ideal for creating variety in the teaching process.

Communication

The ability to communicate well marks the difference between an average and an excellent instructor. As instructors, we need to make communication a top priority. We need to be open to other people and create a receptive environment for communication.

Communication can be defined as the transfer of information from one person to another person, or from one person to a group of people. It is a two-way process, involving the sending and receiving of information. For you, communication occurs before, during and after your class.

Communication can be achieved through three major avenues—verbal, non-verbal and written. Instructors are required to use verbal and non-verbal techniques to perform their role as a group exercise leader. The written form of communication can be used in a circuit-style workout, where cards contain the exercise description or content for participants to follow.

Effective cueing is integral to good communication and, having already covered verbal and non-verbal techniques, it is interesting to note the following statistics:

7%	of communication is done through the use of words;
38%	is from voice intonations;
55%	is from the use of body language, ie. mannerisms, body position, dress, etc.

Therefore, by simply relying on the content of our conversation to create rapport, we miss a large part of creating commonality with other people. Put simply, it is not so much what you say but how you say it, and the way in which your body expresses it, that is going to make a difference in your classes.

Verbal communication

When sending information, the instructor has the role of putting it in a logical order and keeping the listener focused and interested. You have to use terminology that is easily understood and user-friendly. The following highlights the important aspects.

Don't say 'don't'

The use of the word 'don't' tends to have a negative connotation. It is like saying 'No, you are wrong!' Approach each cue or teaching tip with a positive attitude. If you see a member using incorrect form and posture, the best way to get results from that person will be to focus on the positive aspects. Comments such as 'Don't arch your back' should be replaced with such comments as 'Let's hold our abs in tight and keep our backs as straight as possible. Yes, well done'.

Use 'let's', 'we', 'your' and 'our' instead of 'I', 'those' and 'that'. Personalise the workout for your participants. Instead of saying 'Lift those legs', use comments such as 'Lift your legs' or 'Let's lift our legs higher, come on everyone'. Focus on positive terminology.

Pre-class considerations

Most fitness centres have their own guidelines on pre-class requirements for their permanent and freelance aerobics instructors. Most centres require you to arrive at least 15 minutes before the commencement of your class. This will allow you plenty of time to mingle with the participants who are waiting for the class to start. Although you, the instructor, should make the first approach to the participants, many of us find it difficult to both start and exit a conversation with comfort and without offence. By practising and employing the following tactics, you will find it much easier to enter and exit conversations with your participants.

Entering a conversation

Finding the right way to enter a conversation comes with time and practice. Many different cultures approach a greeting or introduction very differently. Most commonly, when trying to commence a conversation there are three ways to begin:
1. ask a question;
2. give an opinion; or
3. state a fact.

This should refer to one of the following topics:
- the situation;
- the other person; or
- yourself.

Remember that either 'the situation' or 'the other person' should always precede comments on yourself. Some of us find it easier to talk about ourselves, especially if we are not overly familiar with the person we are speaking to. But if you are continually making reference to yourself, you will often lose the person's attention or respect. As an instructor you are there to lead the group and make them feel good about themselves from both a personal and a physical perspective.

Introduction of the class

While the pre-class scene is important, the first few minutes of your class will be even more important for creating a professional and caring image in your participants' minds. The introduction of the class is essential, as first impressions do make a difference. Participants will start to form an opinion on what type of person you are and what type of class you will present from the moment you start talking. A script or set introduction should be completed at the start of each and every class as a way of preparing your participants for the workout to come. This is an important part of every class and often it is your first point of communication for the day with many of your participants.

Start the class introduction right on time. It is a necessary part of the class. This will allow for any questions from participants or a quick explanation to newcomers. It will also allow latecomers to do the warm-up. If you are teaching back-to-back classes, still make a few minutes to prepare your participants with an INTRO. A thorough introduction of the class may read as follows:

I	Introduce yourself and greet the class
N	Name the type of class to be taught
T	Talk about the class components
R	Reassure newcomers and first starters
O	Organise the group to commence/organise equipment required.

Try the following introduction for a Step Athletic class, or incorporate it into your existing script:

I Good morning everyone and welcome, my name is ...
N Today's class is a 60-minute Step Athletic class.
T After our warm-up, we will have a section of non-propulsive Step with weights, followed by Power

Step, muscle conditioning and a cool down

R   If you are new to a Step Athletic class, please remember that armlines are optional, as are hand weights. Power Step can also be done without the use of propulsions. Feel comfortable to work at your own pace throughout the class, and take a drink break whenever necessary.

O   If you are using hand weights, please place them under your platform ready for the non-propulsive Step segment. Please position steps with the short ends to the front and back of the room and stand on the left-hand side of the step ready for the warm-up.

To avoid predictability you can shuffle the order of the INTRO, e.g. NRTOI. This will introduce the class, welcome newcomers first and put them at ease at the start of the class.

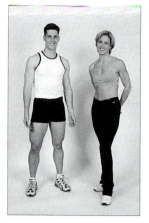 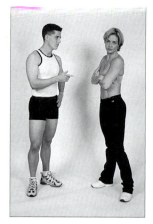

1. Friendly body posture and facial expressions

2. Non-friendly body postures and facial expressions

Fig. 6.1. Body postures and expressions

Drill

Now create your own script for one of the following classes: Hi-Lo, Low Impact, Cross Training.

Non-friendly	Friendly
Frowning	Smiling
Shaking head	Winking
Rolling eyes	Nodding
Looking away	Laughing
Yawning	Eye contact

Non-verbal communication

Non-friendly	Friendly
Pointing	Palms open
Arms crossed	Turn and face
Hands on hips	Open position
Covering your mouth with the microphone	Soft joints
Turning your back while speaking	Hands by your sides
INTRO from behind the step	Feet turned

Table 6.2. Body postures and body expressions

Non-verbal communication is a powerful medium. Without a word from you, your participants will be able to evaluate your motivation level through facial expressions and body positions. Positive body language can mark the difference between an average and a great instructor.

Body language and facial expressions

First impressions do count. When talking, the real meaning behind the words comes from intonation, facial expression and gestures. These expressions and gestures, both friendly and non-friendly, can lead to misinterpretation by your participants (see Table 6.1). Certain body postures are also used and these, too, can be interpreted as being friendly and non-friendly (see Table 6.2). If our goal is to develop rapport, we need to be aware of these important non-verbal messages.

Eye contact

Regular eye contact will make your classes more personal. Instructors whose eyes tend to skim over the heads of their group or, to the other extent, look at their feet, fail to make that special connection. Be aware of your own comfort level when instructing. If your regulars in the front row happen to be the only ones that smile back at you, don't slip into your comfort zone and only look at this group for reassurance. If someone at the back of your group isn't able to get the set routine, then give them a nod also, to acknowledge that everything is OK. The back row of your class generally needs more reassurance. Be sure to look at everyone in your group. It is very motivational to have someone look you in the eye with a friendly facial expression, but avoid the 'death stare'. Participants will respond to this form of communication. A good instructor will try to make eye contact with every participant.

Touching

There are many people who feel very comfortable with touching and being touched by others. There are also people who do not like to be touched, and who feel uncomfortable touching another person. But touching, if done sensitively, can achieve a number of goals and can be a great way of building trust and rapport in your relationships with your participants and with people in general. Touching can not only be reassuring, it can be a simple gesture to let participants know that you haven't forgotten them, and it can break down the barriers between you and another person. Some points of contact are more appropriate than others (see Table 6.3). Learn to distinguish your participants' comfort level and develop your own techniques that both you and your participants are comfortable with before, during and after the classes.

Taboo contact areas Soft points	OK contact areas Hard points
Mid thigh	Knee
Face	Elbow
Abdominals	Shoulder
Gluteals	Foot or shoe

Table 6.3. **Points of contact**

Ranges of personal space

It is easy to pick up an individual's spacial awareness. The amount of personal space that an individual requires will vary from one person to the next. Try to notice how close or how far your participants stand when they speak to you. By keeping the same amount of space between the two of you when you speak, you will avoid encroaching on their personal space. Even as your relationship or rapport develops, it doesn't necessarily mean that the space between you two will change. This spacial awareness, and the comfort level associated with it, will remain fairly constant with each individual. In addition, be aware of your own preferences concerning personal space and, indeed, touching.

Appropriate dress

Dress can create a barrier if participants cannot relate to it. Be mindful of your target audience and dress in a manner that is not intimidating. To set the mood in your classes, try to select your instructor outfit to suit your group. For example, a close fitting and revealing outfit for an over-50s class is not appropriate. A cap may be worn during a kids' class, and a big T-shirt may be worn for a beginners' class. These outfits are both non-threatening and comfortable for all to wear. They allow the participants to relate to the instructor during the class.

Keys to successful communication

Building rapport

Building rapport with your participants is the key to effective communication techniques. Communication is built on trusting relationships. Rapport is the ability to enter another person's world, to make them feel you understand them, that you have a strong common bond. The successful instructor develops an affinity, an understanding and a harmonious inter-relationship with people from all walks of life, irrespective of their differences in background, race or culture. The ability to establish rapport readily and easily is one of the greatest skills a person can have. Having a good understanding of different personality types, including your own, will definitely assist the building of rapport.

Leadership skills

The skills of a leader are developed over a period of time. Some instructors have the ability to feel very comfortable in front of a new group, while others may have to 'warm up' to the group over a period of time. As an instructor, the emphasis is not always on you leading your group for the full 1-hour session, but how you can share the leadership within your group. Simple teaching techniques such as effective planning and different class formats can allow this leadership to be shared amongst your group. The wealth of knowledge and enthusiasm from a group of leaders far outweighs that of one leader. Remember that leadership is not always reserved for people in positions of authority.

The vital first 10 minutes

There are vital times when communication is more important in your classes. One direct example of this is the first 10 minutes of your class, and even the time before your class starts. As an instructor, you must be able to lead the communication competently during the first ten minutes of a class.

When preparing for your class, ensure that you arrive at the fitness club with your music and class plan already formulated. Chat to members as you set up any necessary equipment, and approach any newcomers. New members of the class may need time to feel confident in you and in their own ability to participate in the class level or format. Reassure newcomers and those exercisers who have recently returned to the club after a period of time away. Welcome all of your participants and make them feel comfortable.

Give all the necessary tips or pointers that they may need before they commence exercising. Some of these pointers could include the following comment for a Step class: 'When placing your foot onto the step, ensure that the whole foot is in contact with the step' or 'Armlines are optional and if they make your leg patterns change or stop, then leave the arms by your side until you have mastered the leg patterns'.

Make sure that you walk in and make eye contact with your participants; smile and say 'hello'. Don't just walk in and start to adjust the stereo system or sneak in with your head down. Make a confident and happy entrance—this will set the scene for a great class.

A log book summary (see Appendix II) will assist in your class preparation and will be a great help when you may be running late and your preparation is not what it should be. Start your own file of class plans and this will assist with your continued professionalism.

Pay attention to first-timers

Go through your INTRO script at the start of the class to identify new participants. Do you remember what it felt like the first time you joined an aerobics class, or even how different it felt coming back after a break? You may find that first-timers do not want to identify themselves at the start of the class. As an instructor, you may need to move around the group before you start, and identify any new faces. When doing this, always introduce yourself and ask if they are new to your class, but first turn off your microphone. Make eye contact with your newcomers throughout the class to continually reassure them.

Class conclusion

Always offer your advice and services to the group at the end of a class. Allow time for any additional or individual counselling. Participants need to be educated and will look to you for advice and wisdom. Offer all participants, and especially newcomers, the opportunity to ask any questions regarding the class, future classes or their own workouts. Always carry through with this offer of assistance. Avoid turning your back on the group straight after class, collecting your music and chatting to the next instructor. Quickly move from the stereo system and position yourself closer to your group so that you become more approachable. If the next class starts immediately, you should position yourself by the door.

Motivation

The art of motivation or the ability to motivate a group can be a challenging yet enjoyable task. Motivation involves encouraging yourself or other people to take action. You motivate your participants to do their best and you challenge and assist them in achieving their goals.

Individual motivation comes in two forms. The first is *intrinsic motivation*. This can be best defined as an inner drive, goal or ambition to want to succeed. You do it for yourself, for fun, to feel better about yourself or for the fact that you know it will improve 'you'. Not for anyone or anything else but yourself. As an instructor, try to develop this form of motivation in your participants with such comments as 'Do it for yourself', 'You are the one that can make a difference', or 'Come on, you know how hard you can work'.

The second type of motivation is termed *extrinsic motivation*. Extrinsic motivation is best defined as being inspired or motivated from an external or outside source, e.g. for a reward, trophy, gift, praise, money or material possession or to avoid punishment. In other words, you will do it because you know that you will get something tangible in return for it. Extrinsic motivational comments could include 'The first one finished will receive a free drink' or 'Complete this last set and you can go home and have a treat'. The difference between intrinsic and extrinsic comments is obvious. Ideally, what you want is a group of self-motivated participants. The best type of reward that we can offer to extrinsically motivated people is the gift of health and fitness. Continually reinforce the personal benefits of attending your classes. Remember that no two people are alike. You should attempt to learn which form of motivation drives your group and always vary your comments and motivational techniques.

Use key words and phrases to motivate your group. The human factor is what will keep participants coming back to your classes. Instructors can provide the personality factor and education that exercise equipment cannot. Don't create distance between you and your participants. They will continually look to you for motivation. Encourage greatness, extra effort and enjoyment in class. Work hard to develop rapport with your participants.

As an instructor, you would surely have a repertoire of your own motivating phrases. These are used to inspire and encourage your participants throughout their workouts. Some additional examples of motivational phrases could include:
- Success consists of a series of little daily efforts.
- Goals don't work unless you do.
- You will only get out of it what you put into it.

The best way to find additional motivational phrases is to buy a book of quotes or sporting books such as autobiographies or team novels. This is a great way to keep yourself motivated as well. Practise these phrases before you put them into your classes, so that first you are comfortable with the phrase, and second you ensure that it is recited correctly.

As for yourself, consider the philosophy expressed in *The Leader in You* (1993) by Schwab, Levine and Crom:

> I consider my ability to arouse enthusiasm to be the greatest asset I possess, and I believe the way to develop the best in anyone is by appreciation and encouragement. There is nothing else that kills ambition like criticism from superiors. So I never criticise anyone. I am anxious to praise but slow to find fault. If I like something, I am hearty in my appreciation and lavish in my praise.

Praise and acknowledgment

Praise or progress reminders are an important component of any workout. Everyone, including ourselves, likes to have their efforts acknowledged and to feel that they are achieving. Acknowledgment cues of how participants are performing like 'great', 'that's better alignment', 'well done', 'you're on fire today', 'super effort', 'so much energy', etc. allow participants to feel a part of the group. This type of positive verbal feedback is adequate, but will not be very effective in the long term. Such comments will not be effective at all if they are overused. Positive non-verbal acknowledgments will be more effective, as they are more personalised and genuine. These include smiling, winking and thumbs up for approval.

Positive feedback, specific information and educational content should be utilised when addressing participants. Use such comments as 'That's great form with your squats' or make it even more personalised by saying 'Great technique, Sally'. A person's name is the single most important thing that they can own. Positive feedback with real value will always gain respect and rapport with your participants. Learn your participants' names and use them on occasions. Don't favour one or two participants because you can only remember their names, make a conscious effort to get to know your group and address all participants at some time during classes. 'Progress awareness' is a major factor when it comes to exercise adherence. So let your participants know exactly how they are performing and progressing throughout the class to ensure that they keep coming back for more.

Ensure that you always vary your praise and progress cues. The overuse of words such as 'great' and 'good' can devalue their meaning. In addition, be careful with the standard of the word you use. If you comment that a participant's efforts are excellent, remember that this word is the best that you can do. The word 'excellent' will be the standard for all other participants. They will feel they must strive to match this standard. Be certain that the effort is the best that you have seen performed before you use a word with such a powerful meaning and high standards. Again, if this word is overused, you must have a very high standard of fit participants within your group. Always be genuine and sincere with your praise and progress cues and make sure that the tone of your voice conveys that sincerity.

Interaction through conversation

In your supervisory role as an instructor during classes, it may be difficult to get into a conversation with your participants or one participant. However, a conversation involves provoking a response or an interchange of thoughts. Ideal conversational situations during the class may be the stretch after the warm-up, during the muscle-conditioning phase of the class, the abdominal section, or during the cool-down. Examples of conversation topics or opening lines could include:

- Did anyone go to the movies/see a good video lately? What did you see? How was it? Would you recommend it?
- Is anyone going anywhere different this weekend?
- Who's got a birthday coming up soon?
- Can anyone pick the artist of this song? What is another song they sing?

If you are asking questions to start a conversation, ensure that your questions consider the use of both closed and open questions. Closed questions allow for simple one- or two-word answers, e.g. yes or no. Open questions are up to the interpretation of the person answering and generally require that person to give you a more detailed answer. Closed questions will help to end a conversation well. Open questions will require an additional comment or question from you. Learn to use both styles of questions to your advantage.

Don't limit your conversational subjects in the class just to your workout. Participants will be interested in general knowledge, society and health and fitness related topics. These topics may be introduced at any stage, depending of course on the type of class you are teaching. Less complex classes often lend themselves to comments and throw-away conversational pieces. The more complex the class, the less time you will have to strike up conversations with your group. A class should never be so complex that you can't have fun and communicate!

Any of the following categories may be useful when addressing your group:
- Current affairs
- Movie stars
- Entertainment
- Nutrition
- Environment
- Sport
- Fitness

Education

Your role as an educator should never be underestimated when instructing. By staying continually updated with all of the latest research in our ever-changing industry, you will be a valuable source of knowledge that your participants can draw on at any time before, during and after your classes.

When we educate, we pass on information that is valuable. Always aim to educate your participants throughout your classes. Some simple examples of educational information can include:
- I found a great book that lists all the fat content of just about every food you can think of—if you'd like to check up on your favourites come and see me at the end of the class.
- Here comes a body check—head up, shoulders back, abdominals held tight and make sure your whole foot is stepping onto the platform.
- Short limbs are easier to move than long limbs. So if your arms are long, try this alternative ...

Fit Facts are useful and important information to reinforce a fit and healthy lifestyle. They can be used at any time during your classes. Examples of simple yet effec-

tive Fit Facts include:
- Carbohydrates are easy to digest and by consuming them we can retain a high level of water in the body. What a perfect choice for a snack before a workout.
- Your body needs six to eight glasses of water per day. If you weigh yourself before and after exercise and you have lost weight, that weight loss is water. You need to replace 1 litre of water for every kilogram lost.
- Massage can help increase circulation, prevent or loosen adhesion and induce relaxation. But it has no value in developing physical fitness or in weight loss.

Cue cards

Educational cue cards are designed to offer important educational tips to your participants. To make it easy for you to remember, the facts should be written in point form in a logical order to allow for easy understanding. These cue cards can be useful for delivery during the first stretch after the warm-up, during the muscle conditioning or the cool-down phases of your classes. The following is a list of easily prepared topics and an example of two cue cards to try on your participants:

Fat and cholesterol.	The benefits of exercise.
Caffeine.	The myth of spot reduction.
The benefits of resistance training.	How to choose an exercise video.
Home workouts.	Anti-stress techniques.
Shoe buyer's guide.	How to increase your metabolism.
A balanced diet.	How to lose fat.

The Myth of Spot Reduction
Educational tips:

- **Fat cannot be lost from specific areas of the body simply by exercising that area.**
- **Research shows that fat is reduced from fat stores all over the body as a result of exercise.**
- **To reduce fat from your fat stores, participate in regular aerobic exercise and ensure that your diet is low in fat (maximum 25–30%).**
- **Include resistance training to enhance overall results.**

Caffeine
Educational tips:

- **Caffeine in moderation is not in itself a risk factor. However, the caffeine in coffee, tea and certain other beverages and medicines can increase blood pressure and may cause temporary heart beat irregularities in some people.**
- **It is a good idea to limit your caffeine intake to 250 mg/day or less. One cup of brewed coffee has about 85 mg, instant coffee 60 mg, tea about 50 mg and cola-type soft drinks about 35 mg/can.**
- **Because caffeine is a stimulant, it is banned by the International Olympics Committee. Athletes are not allowed more than 12 mg per litre of urine, which corresponds to about 8 cups of coffee or 16 cans of cola consumed 2–3 hours before competition.**

Humour

Humour can come in many forms. During your class try to use simple forms of humour to capture or enhance the mood and attention of the participants. Simple techniques such as tongue twisters, light humorous jokes or a funny personal story can have positive influences on your classes. Humour can be obtained from short stories, borrowed from books and newspapers and adapted to suit your audience. The daily newspaper will usually have humorous stories to use.

One key to building rapport is to learn to laugh at yourself. If you make a simple cueing or instructional error during your class, always be the first to laugh. This allows participants to feel more relaxed. Create an open and enjoyable atmosphere within your classes to put participants at ease and allow them to enjoy their physical workout.

Always remember that your participants attend your classes for any number of reasons. These could include stress release, escapism, to increase fitness, to improve their physical appearance, social aspects, to release pent-up emotions or energy, and for fun. The instructor who is a 'fun' and supportive person who makes them laugh will always have participants coming back for more.

Mind wake-ups

Mind wake-up drills have always been a valuable part of education experience. It has been proven that such drills can prepare our minds for an event or experience to follow. Mind wake-up drills can be used at the beginning of a class to 'switch on' the minds of participants and get them to focus on you as the group leader. Stimulating their minds before they begin not only leads to better attention in class but also injects some initial energy into the workout.

Workout-related mind wake-ups

- Ask participants to face a particular point or geographic landmark. Verbalise a move and have your participants perform the move.
- Use a body awareness drill, such as 'Put your left foot on the step and cross your right arm over your chest'.
- Ask the group to balance on one foot with their eyes closed for 3 seconds.

Non-workout-related mind wake-ups

- How many I's are contained in the word Mississippi?
- What is the answer to 5 + 9 + 14?
- Play great walk-in music to get your participants in the mood.
- Which is normal/average BP? 150/80?

Handling difficult situations

Unfortunately, instructing is not always smooth sailing. Even after years of experience, you may be faced with many situations that are awkward, embarrassing, hilarious, frustrating, challenging or even impossible. Good communication is essential. Listed below are samples of situations, accompanied by a suggested solution, but before you read these, try the following drill:

⚒ ⚒ Drill ⚒ ⚒

Make a list of the situations listed below and write your own way of handling each one. Compare this with the suggested solution. Your responses are important to ensure you remain both professional and respected as an instructor.

Situation: Beginners arriving late to class.
Suggested solution: Some centres will not allow latecomers to join a class after the warm-up has been completed. Consult your manager for policies. Assistance can be sought from the gym staff with a warm-up and brief class INTRO. If appropriate, advise the 'late' beginner to do low impact for at least 5–10 minutes. Get the class to perform the routine through several times and speak to the newcomer in person with the microphone turned off.

Situation: Dealing with extremely different skill levels in the same class, or where some people pick up routines faster than others.
Suggested solution: Intensity can be used as a tool to divide experienced from less experienced participants. Provide more intense options for the experienced participants. Complexity can also be used to divide skill levels. Offer levels of variation, e.g. Level 1—base move; Level 2—an element of variation, e.g. direction change; Level 3—two or more changes, e.g. armline and travel pattern. Increase your cueing to benefit all participants. This will be great for newcomers, and regulars will appreciate the review.

Situation: You forget the moves or combination you are teaching.
Suggested solution: Use a holding pattern or send class for a power walk or run around the room to allow you time to recall. Alternatively, ask the regulars in a light way, 'Now it's your turn, show me the next move'. This may disguise the fact that you have forgotten and may be used as a participant mind wake-up drill.

Situation: Class participants doing their own thing.
Suggested solution: Increase your cueing, as they may not have heard you. Depending on their position in class, eg. front row vs back or middle of the group, they may or may not disturb other participants. If what they are doing is safe and it is keeping their heart rate up, you may choose to leave them, unless of course their movements are dangerous. Speak with them in private after class to see if you can assist with their class satisfaction level. Perhaps you may need to suggest a different class level or type.

Situation: Class participants talking excessively.
Suggested solution: Don't forget that most of your participants are in class to enjoy themselves and feel good, but if it disturbs others then some humour often helps, e.g. 'You must have had a good weekend'. It may be appropriate to share some good news with the entire group, eg. during warm-up or cool-down or after class. This end-of-class talk may also make the participant aware that their talking may have been a little excessive during the class.

Situation: Someone in the class is criticising what or how you are teaching.
Suggested solution: If they are not disrupting too much, ignore them and deal with it after class. If they are disrupting the class, then suggest discussing it after class and you will gladly comment. Depending on your level of experience, either talk to the manager about your concern or ask the participant to talk to the manager. Evaluate the situation to see if it is a personal attack on your ability, a personality clash, or if your participant is just having a bad day.

Situation: The sound system breaks down.
Suggested solution: Ask staff or management for assistance. Familiarise yourself as to where the spare system is kept and how to operate it. Change your class plan to incorporate a circuit or, depending on the location of the club and the insurance factors, do an outdoor session.

Situation: You forget your music, or a tape breaks without a back-up.
Suggested solution: This situation should rarely occur. A good instructor will always carry spares, and the centre may also. If your tape does break due to the poor quality of the centre's stereo system, speak with the management regarding replacement or repair of the tape.

Situation: Dealing with an injury in class.
Suggested solution: Ideally, if another instructor is available ask them to either deal with the injury or deal with the class while you advise the injured participant. If there is no available instructor, place the class in a holding pattern while you deal with the injury. For serious injuries you may need to terminate the class and deal with the injury. Be aware of where ice and the first-aid box is kept at the centre. Often, the duty managers are qualified to deal with injuries.

Conclusion

If you wish to become a master communicator, you must master many areas. What you say isn't quite as important as your delivery. Practise the different methods of verbal and non-verbal communication. Change your tone of voice, practise your body language, and educate your participants. The greatest tragedy in teaching is knowing your subject matter but not knowing your participants.

Rapport is accessible to all—all you need are your eyes, your ears and your senses. These are tools you already have at your disposal. Rapport doesn't mean just smiling, it means responsiveness! Rapport is not static, it is not stable once it is achieved! Communication is always a two-way process. Always keep your communication channels open to give and receive information and feedback. Really listen and hear your participants. Try to turn conversations around to favour them. Use keen observation and be flexible when dealing with others. Encourage your participants with words of greatness and motivation.

Warm-Ups

When aerobics became popular in the early '80s, very little attention was given to warming up. Participants and instructors wanted to get right into the 'thick of it' and forget about the warm-up, and as a result many unnecessary injuries occurred. To ensure that our industry would be around for the long term, health and fitness professionals worldwide rallied and the war cry became 'Thou Must Stretch'.

This resulted in an improvement in safety, but many participants found the minimum ten minutes of stretching very boring. If flexibility dominates the warm-up, the many other aspects of participant preparation go missing. These include the mental aspects, as well as the physical elements, of the warm-up.

Today's warm-up is both dynamic and stimulating. It provides participants with a good balance of mobility work, physical and mental preparation, and a small amount of flexibility training. The emphasis on flexibility training now occurs during the cool-down phase by the use of static stretches.

Integral components of the modern warm-up

The purpose of the warm-up is to prepare the body for the stress of overload during the conditioning phase of the class, and its importance should not be understated. It is like turning your car on and letting it idle for a short time. The car will always run better when it is warmed up.

The same thing applies to the body. The warm-up can be general and specific and it should take up approximately 10–20% of the total workout time. When planning your warm-up, be certain to include the following.

Warming the body

When body temperature is increased, the soft tissue (muscle and connective tissue) becomes more elastic, thus reducing the potential for strain or injury. The warm-up should stimulate the heart and lungs moderately and the blood flow also increases, enabling more oxygen and energy substrates to be carried to the working parts of the body. Each participant needs to be prepared psychologically for the workout to come. The majority of the exercises in the warm-up should be brisk, rhythmical, compound movements. All muscle groups should be addressed.

Mobility

Mobility involves using a muscle and a joint throughout its range of movement. Many participants have been sitting behind a desk, driving or standing behind a counter for the majority of the day, thus compromising their posture prior to class. This must be corrected and normal range of motion restored to ensure a safe and effective workout. As an aerobics instructor you must consider these factors when planning your afternoon or evening classes. Morning classes should also address postural correctness. This will leave your participants with a positive message to carry with them throughout the day.

Specific stretching

Increasing mobility will generally be achieved through the warming-up exercises. However, some areas of the body need special attention, e.g. calves, hamstrings, lower back and hip flexors. Specific range of motion stretches should be included to target these important areas.

These are the 'bare bones' or the essential stretches for each class, and can be best achieved through dynamic stretching (see Fig. 7.1). Dynamic stretching involves repeated slow, controlled, rhythmical movements throughout the range of motion. Some static stretching —stretching that is held for 10–30 seconds without bouncing—can also be included to complement the dynamic stretching. This is particularly useful for new exercisers, as it allows them to focus on their body alignment and correct form.

It is important to be able to evaluate the needs and wants of the exercising group to determine how much and what type of stretching is required. Class specifics are also a major factor. Ask yourself such questions as 'What major muscle groups will we target in today's class that need particular attention during the warm-up?', or 'Are we using hand-held weights or resistance tubing?', or 'How can I provide a more balanced workout for the muscles in the warm-up?'

Vary the stretches used and/or the transitions used to arrive at the stretch position. Try 'freezing' some movements mid-air or halfway through the completion of a move and then move to your stretch position from this point. This different approach will focus your participants' concentration, balance and posture. An example of this could be a touch step (side). Freeze the touch step at one side with the leg extended. Bend your support leg for balance, lift the outstretched leg in a quarter circle to the rear and then lower the foot and heel of this leg into a standing calf stretch.

Stretches can be interspersed throughout the warm-up, or placed predominantly at the end of the warm-up track. Don't let stretching limit your creativity. Place some additional moves in between stretching either the left or right legs, and keep the momentum of your warm-up going.

Listed below is an example of a warm-up static/dynamic stretch combination. 'Dynamic' refers to range of motion or movement about the joints. The static stretch is a fixed joint stretch, held without bouncing for 10–30 seconds. No stretch should be held for more than 30 seconds during the warm-up, as this would interrupt the physical benefits of the warm-up by keeping the class stationary for additional time.

The delivery of your warm-up must be accompanied by the right balance of 'mobility' and 'warming-up' exercises, as well as an enjoyable format. Make sure you supply great music!

Static/dynamic stretch sequence
Starting position: facing front feet together.
- Reverse ezy walk R x 4 (step bwd first).
- Take the first step in the reverse easy walk R and hold *hamstring stretch* L.
- Tap L toe x 4, clap hands on count 4, and repeat.
- Place both hands on L thigh and roll up into a *lower back stretch*.
- Shift body weight onto L leg in lunge position. Lift and lower R heel off ground x 8 (counts 1–16) for dynamic *calf stretch* R.
- Shift body weight further onto L leg hold R foot in R hand for *hip flexor/quad stretch* R.
- Repeat the above steps starting with L leg.

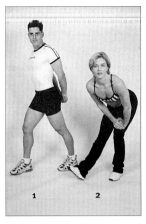

1. Compound calf/pectoral
2. Standing hamstring
3. Standing lower back
4. Standing hip flexor

Fig. 7.1. **The 'bare bones' or essential stretches**

Considerations for the warm-up

While the major components of the modern warm-up are accepted among fitness professionals in the industry, problems still exist with the specific content of many warm-ups. Your participants will know what a great warm-up feels like. Learn from their satisfaction levels and try to avoid making some of the most frequent errors. Some important considerations are:

Starting the warm-up

As the group leader it is important to know that the warm-up always begins before and not after the music starts. It is essential to welcome the participants, both newcomers and regulars, with your INTRO (see Chapter 6).

Music selection

Listen to your music before the commencement of the class. The warm-up track must be inspiring and motivating. An inappropriate selection of warm-up music can affect the remainder of the class. The selected music must suit the style of workout, as well as the participants' age and experience level. Don't give your over-50s class the latest funk music; hits from the 1960s are far more appropriate.

Incorrect speed

This can either make the warm-up unexciting and tedious or super-fast, which is not only ineffective but can also cause injuries. The current acceptable range for a safe and effective warm-up for a standard Hi-Lo class is 130–138 bpm. Don't be misled into thinking that increasing music speed is the only way to increase exercise intensity. As an instructor, you only have your participants to answer to after each class—you should not try to impress your peers or colleagues by increasing the music speed. The guidelines are there as a tool for you to use and follow for reasons of safety, range of movement ease and effectiveness. Follow the guidelines and strive for professionalism.

Impact

Low- or non-impact moves should be used in the warm-up. Using airborne moves in this early stage of the workout generally increases the risk of injury. If you are teaching a multi-impact class, then ease into the varying levels of impact through the conditioning phase. The occasional use of a moderate-impact move in the warm-up may be necessary to enable a safe change in direction or change in lead leg, but these are more soundly integrated after the tissues of the feet and lower leg are adequately prepared. Even if you are aware that several of your participants have already warmed up before your class, don't let these few participants dictate the style of your warm-up. Always cater for the majority of your group, and if a participant does come late and misses the warm-up phase of the class, have them keep their impact to a minimum until they are sufficiently warmed up.

Overhead armlines

These actions are permitted, but overuse should be avoided during the initial stages of the warm-up. This is recommended due to the fact that an increased strain is placed on the circulatory system through the transportation of blood to areas above the level of the heart. In unfit members this may increase breathing and heart rate quite rapidly. Further, overuse or continual targeting of the deltoid muscle group is not advised due to the fact that this is one area that is predominantly used in the workout phase. Developing unnecessary fatigue in this area at such an early stage is not advisable. Smooth-flowing armlines are also more advisable than sharp, jerky movements. Aim for complementary armlines and foot patterns and introduce more complex armlines slowly.

Stretch positions

Positions requiring participants to lie or sit on the floor should be used sparingly in warm-ups, as they tend to decrease motivation levels and are often too time consuming. Make maximum use of the standing position—your stretches should be designed and incorporated to reflect this upright position. Always stretch the muscles required and then move on to the cardiovascular phase of your workout. Don't get carried away with excessive stretching and lose the momentum or intensity you have created with your warm-up.

Alignment errors

When stretching, ensure that your demonstration and technique is always accompanied by good form and effective cueing. The use of imagery will assist your participants to a better understanding of the stretch and the best position for its execution. Such key words as 'slowly', 'sit back', 'head up', 'hip forward', 'bend your supporting leg' and other phrases will all be useful.

Alignment errors often occur in stretches and, as a consequence, the desired outcome is not achieved. Keep changing your position when demonstrating a stretch. Turn side on, front on or place your back to the group to give them the best view of the stretch involved. Don't feel that you must always face your group. Leading by good example is always an effective way to get the message across.

Complexity

The issue of complexity seems to be on every instructor's lips. How much complexity is enough, or too much? Any combination of moves should be accompanied by the appropriate learning curves and teaching techniques. The warm-up should be designed to meet participants' psychological and physiological needs.

Avoid trying to go for the 'wow' factor in your warm-up. An understanding of the balance between a psychologically uplifting warm-up, a motivating warm-up, and an overly complex one needs to be considered and achieved. Use smart, 'wake-up' choreography that tests the waters of your group's ability level, but remember that overuse of elaborate combinations, armlines and co-ordination type movements usually leads to frustration and inefficient preparation for the workout. Assess each group before and during the delivery of your warm-up. As the instructor, you must be able to accurately monitor your participants' needs, wants and ability levels. If in doubt, you are better to make your warm-up too simple rather than too complex.

Variety

In the quest for an effective and enjoyable warm-up, the element of variety can be achieved in many ways. Aim to include a variety of starting moves, e.g. walking, squatting, step touch, touch step and others. In addition, use a range of teaching methods for your warm-ups, e.g. linear progression vs add on.

Changing the directions you face throughout your warm-up may be a common theme to develop throughout the class. A different direction can totally alter the perception and feel of a workout.

Consider organising your participants into different formations. Avoid the clutter of bodies at the back of the room and try out new shapes such as a circle, a square, lines, two subgroups facing each other or facing the front, etc. You can even alter your teaching position from the front to the back of the room, so that the last person in each line or group now becomes the new leader.

Stationary vs travelling moves

Throughout the warm-up, select a combination of travelling and stationary moves. Start on the spot and gradually incorporate large travel patterns to assist with warming up the body.

You can also trace a variety of shapes on the aerobics floor through the use of travel and direction. The use of floor space will increase the intensity of the warm-up and allow the participants to maximise the area in which they are working.

Remember that it is also comforting to many participants to maintain an element of predictability or consistency. This could be anything from that march at the start of class to the big, deep breath after the stretch. Be aware of your habits when instructing, and learn the comfort zones of your group. The warm-up needs to be

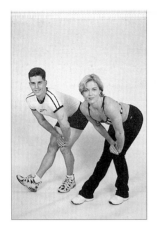
1. Hamstring stretches

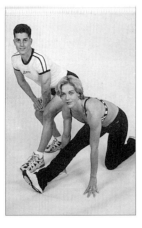
2. Hamstring stretches

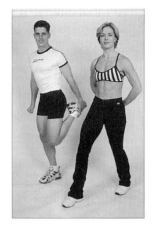
3. Hip flexor stretches

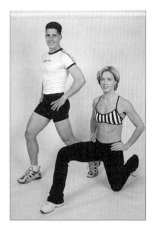
4. Hip flexor stretches

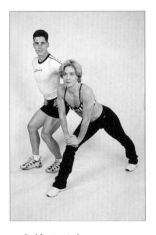
5. Calf stretches

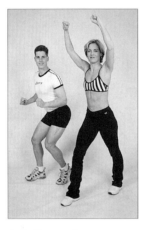
6. Calf stretches

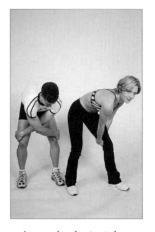
7. Lower back stretches

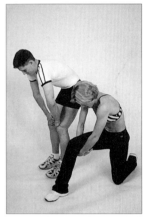
8. Lower back stretches

Fig. 7.2. **Variation stretches**

fun and exciting. The first 10 minutes will set the scene for the rest of your class.

Specific warm-ups

Warm-ups for some workouts may require you to target different muscle groups or to adopt a particular style or sequence of moves in preparation for the workout to follow. The variety of class styles will dictate both your warm-up style, armline and movement selection. The class formats to consider will include weighted workouts, newcomers' or beginners' classes, and specific stylised workouts.

Weighted workouts

Resistance-orientated moves may be inserted into the warm-up to directly reflect the type of activities you will perform in class. Right from the start there should be an emphasis on stronger armlines, controlled movements, range of movement and good form. This will prepare your participants for the class in body and mind.

By including more specific upper body stretches such as deltoids, latissimus dorsi, trapezius and rhomboids, participants can be better prepared for the weighted workout. A combination of both stationary and travelling moves should be included in the warm-up. Such stationary moves may be lunges, squats and lift moves. Travelling moves include grapevines and walking forwards and backwards. Music with a strong, powerful beat should be selected.

New exercisers

Class design for new exercisers should always be slower than for regular classes. All learning curves should be extended due to the fact that new exercisers may not know the exercise vocabulary and may need ample time to pick up the moves that match the names. The group will comprise participants of different age groups, fitness, ability and experience levels. Read the group's warning signs very early and ensure that your cueing emphasises educational tips, correct technique and alignment when stretching.

Keep offering modifications or move sequences that do not include armlines. This will ensure that the leg patterns will be accomplished and the physical components of the warm-up are being met.

Most exercises should be repeated without causing excess isolation and fatigue. Limit the use of any complex combinations or compound movements that require a high level of commitment and co-ordination. Organise your group early so that all participants have a clear view of you at the start of the class. Your group needs to leave at the end of the workout feeling that they have achieved and accomplished in class, rather than feeling frustrated or that they have failed.

The music speed you select may be at the lower end of the recommended speed. Base moves should be selected and you can test your group in the warm-up by adding one or two elements of variation. Ensure that you are well prepared to teach this class.

Stylised workouts

As each new style of class will have a different mood or setting, your warm-up should reflect this 'feel'. The choice of different music will certainly reflect your move selection. All base moves will be modified to suit the class format. If you are using equipment such as steps in your class, this may be incorporated into the warm-up also. Your INTRO should give your participants a good idea of what type of class will follow, and your warm-up will definitely reflect this style. The warm-up will allow the participants to decide if they are going to commit themselves to the class or choose another activity within your centre.

Generally, a stylised workout is one that takes moves from street dance or modern dance classes and incorporates them into the aerobics class. The most common forms on aerobic timetables are Cardio Funk, City Jam and Body Beat classes.

Common warm-up methodologies

The following methods range from freestyle warm-ups to structured warm-ups where combinations are developed. As you learn and understand each method, there will be numerous variations that you can add to each method using your own style, comfort level and personality.

Freestyle
- Linear progression.
- Add and substract, or 'top 'n tail' method.

Combinations
- Add-on method
- Link method

Linear progression is particularly useful, as you only make one change at a time. A variation is called the 'zig-zag' technique, which involves making your way up the ladder in the linear progression to a certain point. At this point the sequence is then put into reverse order and you climb back down the ladder, repeating all changes in reverse order. You can then progress back up the ladder.

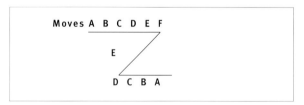

Fig. 7.3. **Zig-zag**

✗ ✗ Drill ✗ ✗

Choreograph a linear progression for the warm-up and include a stretching sequence for the four Bare Bones stretches.

Warm-up concepts

OTS (on the spot)

All movements are done within your immediate personal space. The element of travel is limited and participants can focus on their form, posture and the task at hand without worrying about travelling and having others travel close to them. The lack of travel patterns may cause a decrease in intensity levels. Simple base moves that can be used for an OTS warm-up include: touch steps (side, front, back, heels) and step-touch with simple arm patterns and/or variations.

Right and left balance

The introduction of Step has made us aware of the importance of maintaining equal balance between left and right lead legs. The benefits have now carried over to the aerobic and muscle-conditioning phases of the workout, with many instructors making a conscious effort to balance many of their combinations. This does not include using equal sides of the body, as this has always been taught to achieve balance—it specifically refers to equal use of both right and left lead legs. The use of a neutral move at the end of a combination is one simple way to assist you in changing your lead leg between combinations. Many other techniques exist, such as rhythm changes, single, single and double moves, and weight-bearing to non–weight-bearing moves, or vice versa.

When teaching your combinations, don't automatically assume that your participants will be able to perform the combination to equal standard on their left leg if you normally teach using a right leg lead. Whenever you change the lead leg in your combination, always spend time to develop the combination on the new lead leg. This ensures success for your participants. This is a whole new side of their body and they need to be able to re-learn the combination on this new lead leg.

Even with your advanced groups, repeat each section of the combination in full before adding the elements of variation or decreasing the repetitions of the combination.

Ricochet

This is an enjoyable and fun option to add to any warm-up. With the ricochet method, base moves and variations are joined together using either add-on, link or other previously covered methods and then the sequence is alternately started by sub-groups at different times.

In class, split your group into four subgroups and teach the combination listed below. When the combination has been repeated several times and the participants are competent at performing it, start the ricochet method. Put all groups into a holding pattern until your are ready to cue the start. Ensure that you give your class a precise and simple description of what is expected of them.

Group 1 will start with Move A on your cue at the start of a new block. When Move A is completed, Group 1 will now be onto Move B. Group 2 will start Move A as soon as Group 1 finishes Move A. When Group 2 has finished Move A, they move on to Move B and Group 3 starts Move A. When Group 3 has finished Move A the final subgroup, Group 4, will start Move A. On each new phrase, the next group will start the next move (i.e. every 8 counts). The fun and games begin when each group tries to keep the ricochet going.

Count	Move	Lower Body	Travel	Direction
1–8	A	4 x step touches R, L, R, L	OTS	Face front
1–8	B	2 x march 1, 2, 3, tap 4	FWD/BWD	Face front
1–8	C	2 x ezy walk R	OTS	Face front
1–8	D	4 x squats (legs together)	OTS	Face front
Repeat combination on a left leg lead.				

Cool-Downs

Take your participants on a journey of stretching and relaxation with creative and thorough cool-downs. A thorough cool-down will always involve components of flexibility, stretching, relaxation work and participant education. Effective instruction of cool-downs will assist participants in preventing injury, restoring full range of motion, and developing flexibility via stretching.

The aerobics class is only complete when the cool-down has been performed, and no sooner. How many times have you seen an instructor put on the cool-down music and a large number of participants leave the class? Educate your participants seriously about the importance of the cool-down and encourage them with positive reinforcement.

The cool-down model

An effective cool-down will involve four phases:

1. Recovery	3. Relaxation
2. Flexibility	4. Education

Phase 1 — Recovery

Recovery is an important component of your class. It is performed at the end of the cardiovascular phase of your class or muscle-conditioning phase of the workout. A post-aerobic cool-down involves partial recovery, and the post muscle-conditioning cool-down involves total recovery. Recovery is best accomplished by a continuation of the cardiovascular or muscle-conditioning phases at a decreased intensity level. Quite simply, the previous routine can be performed at a decreased speed and intensity level. This can also be carried out by performing rhythmical movements similar to the warm-up or by performing isolation floor exercises.

There are various reasons for not suddenly ceasing an activity at the end of the cardiovascular or muscle-conditioning phase of the workout. When exercise is terminated suddenly blood tends to 'pool' in the legs and other regions where the muscles have been working. If a cool-down has not taken place, insufficient blood is returned to the heart, which can result in nausea, fainting and dizziness.

The recovery phase helps return the body to a resting state and removes waste products. It will also help prevent cramps, stiffness and muscle soreness, and assists participants to overcome fatigue and exhaustion. During the recovery phase, the exercise intensity level should decrease to a point where flexibility and relaxation exercises are the only focus.

Phase 2 — Flexibility

Flexibility work is essential after the recovery phase. Stretches should incorporate all major muscle groups, with emphasis on those most relevant to the workout and those that tend to be tight.

Stretching is defined as tissue elongation from a resting level. It is normally the method used to improve flexibility. There are three types of tissue involved in the stretching process: muscles, connective tissue (mainly fascia), and other tissues (tendons and ligaments). Without stretching, muscles and connective tissue tend to lose their suppleness. Fitness instructors should not be concerned with increasing the flexibility of tendons and ligaments.

Correct stretching attempts to:
- lengthen muscle and connective tissue;
- reduce muscle tension and therefore increase relaxation;
- prevent traumatic injuries;
- promote blood circulation; and
- enhance performance.

Factors that limit flexibility are:
- joint structure;
- adipose tissue;
- skin;
- gender;
- inflammation or fluid retention;
- muscle temperature;
- muscle bulk;
- fascia;
- age;
- activity level;
- restricted circulation; and
- muscle reflexes.

How to stretch

Stretching should be relaxed and sustained, with the focus on the muscle group being stretched. Remember that the muscles must be warm prior to stretching. There are three main types of stretching:

1. Dynamic stretching. Controlled dynamic stretching techniques can be useful if administered correctly. There are three types of dynamic stretching:

i) Range of motion (ROM) stretching. This is a continuum from gentle to forceful range of movement. The stretch reflex may be initiated but, as this is generally a gentle and slow stretch, the reaction is minimal. This style of stretching is acceptable in an aerobic warm-up and cool-down.

ii) Ballistic stretching. Fast movement takes the joint to a forced range of movement. Momentum is used to achieve this level, therefore the stretch reflex is quite strong. This type of stretching is not acceptable in aerobics.

iii) Bounce stretching. Whereas ballistic stretching generally refers to a single movement, bounce stretching refers to taking the muscle to its end point of ROM and bouncing there. Here the stretch reflex is continually activated and, as a consequence, an individual is trying to elongate the muscle/tissue when it is shortening, leading to muscle tears. Again, this is not acceptable in aerobics.

2. Static stretching. This involves taking the muscle to a position of stretch where it is held, without bouncing, for 10–30 seconds. The feeling of mild tension experienced at this level should subside within the duration of the stretch. This feeling of tension is caused by the initiation of the stretch reflex, a protective mechanism to prevent over-stretching, which causes a muscle contraction as the muscle length is increased. Usually a time period greater than 10 seconds will induce the inverse stretch reflex—when a degree of tension is built up in the muscle through contracting or stretching the muscle, the inverse stretch reflex will cause the muscle to relax to avoid possible rupturing, which allows further lengthening.

3. PNF stretching. PNF stands for proprioceptive neuromuscular facilitation. It is a form of static stretching that incorporates an isometric contraction of the muscle being stretched. An isometric contraction is one where the muscle contracts without moving the joint. This helps stretch the muscle further by making the inverse stretch reflex increase its response, causing greater muscle relaxation. Overall, PNF stretching is the most effective method of increasing flexibility and can be performed either individually or with a partner. However, it is not the most time-efficient method, and this is an important consideration when instructing aerobics classes.

There are two types of PNF stretching:

i) Contract-relax stretch. The technique involves taking the muscle to a position of stretch and then an isometric contraction is completed for 6–8 seconds. The muscle then relaxes and is placed on stretch again by moving into a new position. This procedure is repeated three or four times.

ii) Contract-relax with agonist contraction stretch. This involves the same steps as above but, rather than passively moving to a new stretch, you contract the opposite muscle (agonist) to move into the new position. This method involves the reciprocal inhibition reflex, which causes the muscle to relax even more. The reciprocal inhibition reflex is added to the inverse stretch reflex, resulting in maximal relaxation of the muscle.

Six hints for effective stretching in the cool-down

i) Length of time to hold the stretch. 10–15 seconds is the minimum, and can be extended up to 30 seconds. Continually educate your participants on this time requirement.

ii) Create ideal conditions. Attempt to set the scene. Dim the lights, lower the music volume in your area and lower air conditioning. A lower, slower and softer voice will also create an ideal atmosphere for the cool-down.

iii) Enhance muscle relaxation. Muscle relaxation will enhance your participants' ability to stretch. Additional relaxation techniques could include rubbing the stretched muscle or applying self-massage to the muscle being stretched.

iv) Rotate the limb in the stretched position. Slightly vary the angle of the stretch by rotating the limb in the stretched position. This will effectively stretch all fibres (i.e. medial and lateral components of the muscle).

v) Avoid weight bearing on the muscles being stretched. Effective stretching is only possible when the muscle is relaxed. A prime example of this is a standing hamstring stretch (see the essential stretch cool-down on p. 74). Hands should be placed on the bent leg to support body weight, rather than on the outstretched leg. The weight on the support leg will allow the hamstring stretch to be effective as there is no weight being applied to the stretched leg.

vi) Music selection. A change in the music speed can indicate to your participants that the cool-down has arrived. Select a piece of music that can positively induce relaxation. Avoid overuse of one cool-down tape. Surprise your participants with good variety, e.g. easy listening instrumental or vocal.

Phase 3 — Relaxation

While recovery and flexibility have a high priority, the cool-down also offers additional opportunities for mental, emotional and physical relaxation. It is a stage in the workout when you can capture the attention of every participant. This stage of the cool-down can be enhanced in the following ways:

- Positive reinforcement of your participants' efforts and achievements during the class should be included at this time.

- Progressive relaxation technique can be used effectively to relax both the mind and the body. This can easily be performed by imagery and muscle tension followed by periods of muscle relaxation. Tell participants to count to five, and at each count they increase the contraction of a particular muscle. At the count of five the muscle group will be maximally contracted. Use the visual colour of red to heighten the contraction. Then guide them to progressively relax that same muscle as you count them back to zero or white. The count of zero registers the most relaxed state the muscle has ever been in—remind them that it now 'feels like jelly'.

- Listen to their breathing whilst lying peacefully on the floor. Have participants focus on deep breaths and listen to themselves breathe in and out. This activity can be enhanced by adding a visualisation and can be complemented by a sound-effects tape of either the ocean, whales or the forest.

- The instructor's voice should be perceived as relaxed. Try lowering your volume and tone and slow down your pitch. Use positive and friendly words that will make participants comfortable and relaxed.

Phase 4 — Education

The cool-down is your best chance to educate your members. They should now be relaxed and feeling good. Some ideas for this stage of the cool-down include:

- Inform members on the benefits of cooling down and stretching.
- Encourage the participants to drink fluid after the class to become re-hydrated.
- Make sure your participants have suitable clothes to put on after the class, especially if it is a cold or windy day outside.
- Let them know when you are teaching your next class.
- Give them some information on your club's social activities, such as a party, new class format or a new instructor.
- Leave them with a joke, a health tip or a thought-provoking statement.
- Invite them to stay behind to ask any questions.

The education phase gives you a great opportunity to show your participants that you care about their general wellbeing. The combination of educating and caring for your participants will certainly help build rapport and encourage them to come back again—class number retention is one of the aerobics instructor's key performance indicators.

Cool-down variations — Practical applications

A variety of cool-down routines are outlined in the photos below. Depending on your position at the conclusion of your class, these routines can be easily and effectively used to enhance the flow of the cool-down.

The essential stretch cool-down

This is a time-efficient cool-down. It is used when you only have a small amount of time for this phase of the class (e.g. a 30-minute class) or when you are running out of time. Little or no rhythmic transitional moves are used and only priority areas of the body are stretched. Priority areas should include: calves, hip flexors, hamstrings, lower back and pectorals. Compound stretches are also used to maximise effectiveness of the time available. Specific stretches utilised in the demonstration routine are the bare bones—see Figs. 8.1 (standing routine) and 8.2 (floor routine).

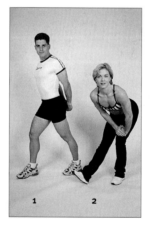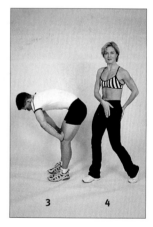

1. Compound calf/pectorals
2. Hamstring
3. Lower back
4. Standing hip flexor

Fig. 8.1. **Bare bones stretches: standing routine**

Basic comprehensive (4–5 minutes)

As more time is available, stretches for the areas outlined above are covered, as well as incorporating additional stretches for the tibialis anterior, gluteals, adductors and upper back. However, little or no rhythmic transitional moves are used. Specific stretches that can be utilised in this routine are illustrated in Fig. 8.3.

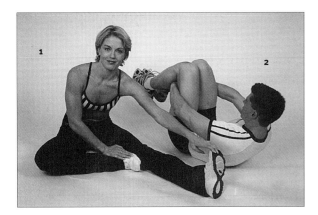

1. Seated hamstring/calf. 2. Lower back

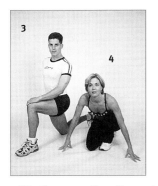 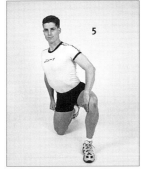

3 Hip flexor. 4 Kneeling soleus 5. Kneeling pectorals

Fig. 8.2. **Bare bones stretches: floor routine**

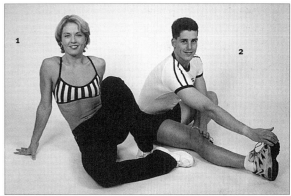

1. Tibialis anterior 2. Soleus/gastrocnemius

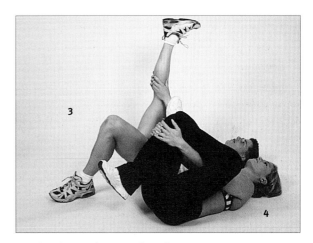

3. Lying hamstring. 4. Gluteal

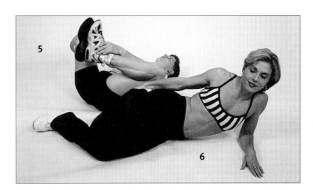

5. Adductor 6. Quadriceps

Fig. 8.3. **Basic comprehensive**

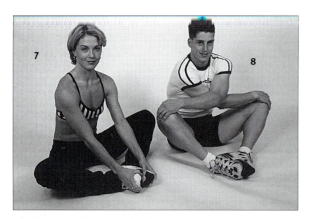

7. Adductor   8. Upper back

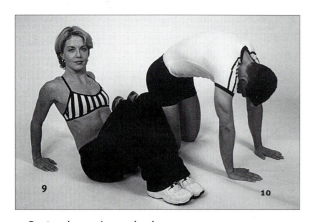

9. Pectoral   10. Lower back

Fig. 8.3 (continued). **Basic comprehensive**

Rhythmic comprehensive (5–0 minutes)

During this cool-down, stretches for the areas outlined in the basic comprehensive method are utilised, but they are interspersed with rhythmic transitions and mobility exercises. The illustrations in Fig 8.4 show specific stretches utilised in this routine.

> ✂ ✂ **Drill** ✂ ✂
>
> Learn and competently demonstrate two cool-down routines that include:
> ✂ post aerobic/recovery phase;
> ✂ flexibility development;
> ✂ relaxation/education.

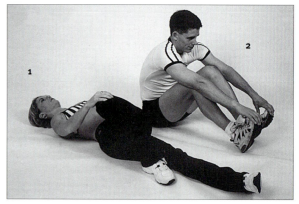

1. Abductor   2. Lower back

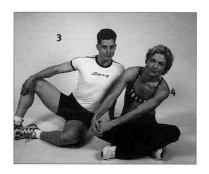

3. Pectoral   4. Upper back/lats

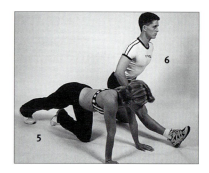

5. Calf   6. Hamstring

Fig. 8.4. **Rhythmic comprehensive**

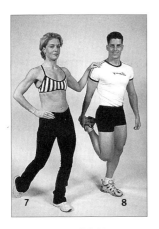
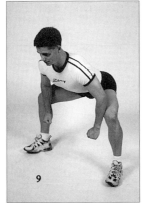

7. Standing tibialis
8. Standing quadriceps
9. Standing adductor

Figure 8.4. (continued) **Rhythmic comprehensive**

Specialty cool-downs

These can include partner cool-downs or partner-assisted specific stretches, or cool-downs that have a theme, e.g. funk. Try to incorporate movements and styles from other cultures, sports or practices. Specialty cool-downs provide a different focus for your participants, adding the elements of fun and enjoyment. The end of the class is the last impression the participants take with them from their workout. Attempt to provide a high point of interest or a new element of variety for the end of your classes, so that you leave your group on a real high.

Special cool-down considerations

Equipment-based classes

After using hand-held weights, barbells or rubberised resistance, more emphasis will be placed on the upper body muscle groups during the cool-down. Specific areas such as the deltoid, pectoral and upper back regions will be targeted for stretching, relaxation and mobility work. Slow ROM or mobility work can be used around the joints of the upper body, arms and shoulders prior to stretching. This will increase the blood flow around the joint prior to the stretch.

Pregnancy

Throughout each stage or trimester in pregnancy, your prenatal participants will be affected by the hormone relaxin, which will affect the elasticity of the ligaments. Special care should be taken to avoid hypermobility during pregnancy.

During pregnancy, prone positions (lying face down) are uncomfortable when attempting stretches. Alternative positions should be instructed or alternative stretches administered.

Supine positions (lying face up) can lead to circulatory problems, due to the weight of the developing baby pressing on the inferior vena cava, the main vein returning the blood from the lower body back to the heart. A decreased blood supply to the uterus can occur in a supine pregnant participant—extreme care should be taken with stretches performed in this position. Specific stretches for the adductors and gluteals are encouraged to assist with labour and delivery. Another consideration is that time and effort are involved when the pregnant exerciser rises from this position.

Body positions for the elderly

There are many considerations when working with elderly participants. Balance is a key issue and the use of a prop such as a wall, step platform, chair or bar can be useful. Try to incorporate non–weight-bearing stretches. PNF stretches should be avoided due to the adverse effect they may have on blood pressure. Obesity may be a concern for some elderly participants. Ensure that seated or lying stretches are modified to facilitate ease of execution of the required stretch.

Kids' fitness

Children are flexible, active and mobile. Ensure that you always place emphasis on teaching both correct technique and breathing. Encourage their efforts as they stretch, and always place emphasis on the importance of stretching. This message of stretching and cooling down is one that they may carry with them for the rest of their lives.

Principles of Muscle Conditioning

The benefits of muscle conditioning both complement and enhance aerobic training. Muscle conditioning or resistance exercise will improve body composition, provide muscular balance and create better general and specific endurance. In addition to this, muscle conditioning or resistance exercise will aid in increasing bone strength, bone density, metabolic rate and enhance physical appearance. Through the use of a load or type of resistance, improvements can be noted in a muscle's condition, including strength, appearance and performance.

The core principles for working with resistance in the aerobics environment involve using body weight, light weights, rubberised equipment or other mechanical methods.

The skill of using body weight as a resistance in the muscle-conditioning component of a class will be examined more closely in this chapter. The instructor's role includes the effective sequencing, planning and putting into action of muscle-conditioning choreography using body weight only. This involves choreography for three key areas: the upper body, the mid-section (core), and the lower body. Muscle-conditioning techniques can be used as a specialised class, such as Body Sculpt, a segment of a class such as Cross Training or Interval, or at the conclusion of a standard aerobics class.

Today muscle conditioning does not only consist of floor work. All the exercises traditionally performed on the floor have made their way into an upright position, which is considered more functional where stabilisation and balance can be incorporated. In addition, more body weight can be utilised, which increases the heart rate during these exercises, and thus the intensity of the workout.

Despite the constant attempts of instructors to educate and inform their participants on the benefits and theories behind muscle conditioning, there still seem to be a lot of myths and misinformation. How many times do we have members ask us questions because they have read an article in the latest women's magazine or in the local paper? Your role as an instructor is to educate your participants so they can make informed decisions directly related to their knowledge. This knowledge is then applied to their own workouts and goals.

Myths and misinformation

The following are common myths and misinformation relating to muscle conditioning:

Pain and gain. The old saying 'No pain, no gain' was a common part of the fitness boom of the early '80s. However, this myth was exploded as instructors and participants alike were introduced to the benefits of cross training and muscle conditioning. Muscle conditioning works on the principle of overload. Overload will create a certain degree of necessary physical discomfort, but discomfort does not mean unbearable pain. Creating participant awareness in regards to the types of pain they will experience is an essential part of muscle conditioning and any resistance program.

Resistance builds bulk. Many participants believe that using resistance such as body weight, tubing, hand weights or even gravity will create a bulky, muscular appearance. The high repetition and low weight nature of resistance classes will never fit into this description. There is a direct relationship between the strength a muscle has and its size. The best way to build size and strength is to use heavy resistance and do fewer repetitions.

Spot reduction. Participants may mistakenly believe that they can lose fat in a given area by performing muscle-conditioning exercises that target that specific spot on the body. It is still common for participants to think that great amounts of localised conditioning work around so-called 'problem areas' of hips, thighs, buttocks or abdominals will promote the loss of body fat in this region. The exercises will work the muscle, but it is aerobic exercise in combination with resistance exercise and a diet low in fat that will promote fat loss.

Line of pull. When planning for effective class cueing and participant education, ensure that you are labelling exercises correctly and focusing on the effects of gravity. An understanding of 'line of pull' is vital for correct exercise analysis. For example, performing a standing pec dec with hand weights is not an effective exercise for the chest, as the movement is not against gravity. In fact, the shoulder and biceps experience most of the load.

Instructor's role in muscle conditioning

- Establish a strong mind–muscle connection through the use of imagery, cueing, descriptive terms, an athletic emphasis and a strong educational focus.
- It is important to consider the general profile of your muscle-conditioning participants. They may be anything from athletes looking for a varied training method to individuals looking for very quick results. They may be overweight, predominantly female and in the 25–40-year age group. A range of alternatives will help cater for everyone.
- Teach correct foot, knee, pelvic and spinal alignment and encourage body awareness. Always offer easier and harder variations and continually emphasise correct body alignment. In addition to this, screen for correct alignment with weight-bearing changes.
- Choose exercises that balance the agonist and antagonist muscle groups. Strategically sequence muscle groups with an attempt to minimise time and maximise fatigue. Create intensity with the basic principles of muscle conditioning, including concentric, eccentric and isometric muscle contractions. Incorporate the stabilisers to enhance safety and muscle control and avoid momentum.
- Essential factors within this class are rest and recovery, which can be achieved with bouts of stretching. Consider the strength and flexibility of your participants and teach control with every exercise.

Muscle-conditioning terms

Agonist: A muscle that is directly engaged in contraction and is the prime mover in a given movement.

Antagonist: A muscle that has the opposite action to the agonist, or prime mover, and in a given movement must relax or lengthen.

Compound movements: Movements that involve more than one muscle or muscle group, and movement at two or more joints.

Concentric contraction: The working of a muscle against gravity, causing a shortening of muscle fibres.

Eccentric contraction: The lowering of a body part assisted by gravity, causing lengthening of muscle fibres.

Isolation movements: Movements that involve a single muscle or muscle group in the action, usually involving movement at one joint only.

Isometric contraction: The working of a muscle where there is no movement with or against gravity and no change in the length of the muscle fibres.

Muscular endurance: The capacity of a muscle to exert force repeatedly over time. It is possible to increase endurance without affecting strength.

Muscular power: The rate or speed that a force can be exerted over a distance.

Muscular strength: The maximum force that can be exerted by a muscle against a resistance. It is possible to increase strength and endurance.

Resistance training: The use of any load that restricts normal movement, generally used to increase gains in muscular strength, power or endurance.

Tone: A marketing term used to describe the appearance and feel of worked muscles. It generally applies to a combination of muscular strength, endurance and definition. Avoid using this term too loosely! Muscle conditioning is a much more appropriate educational term than 'tone'. Other marketing terms may include 'shape up' and 'firm'.

Muscles	Comments/needs	Balance checklist		
		L	M	I
Upper body				
Biceps	Hard to overload without specific use of equipment.	❏	❏	❏
Triceps	Worked via movement at shoulder and elbow.	❏	❏	❏
Deltoid	Overall balance achieved by working through a variety of planes. Tends to be overused.	❏	❏	❏
Trapezius	Mainly involved in movements of the shoulder girdle, which can be tight and in need of stretching.	❏	❏	❏
Rhomboids	Underworked, hard to isolate without equipment and the right body position.	❏	❏	❏
Pectorals	Hard to work in standing position without specific equipment.	❏	❏	❏
Latissimus dorsi	Be wary of line of pull, usually requires a specific position and equipment.	❏	❏	❏
Core				
Rectus abdominus	Weak in most participants. Requires specific attention in almost every class type.	❏	❏	❏
Erector spinae	Quite often weak and tight and should be included when doing abdominal exercise.	❏	❏	❏
Gluteals	Extend the hip and lower back via movements at pelvis.	❏	❏	❏
Iliopsoas (hip flexor)	Generally considered to be tight and strong enough for everyday activities.	❏	❏	❏
Obliques	External and internal obliques worked through spinal rotation and lateral flexion.	❏	❏	❏
Transverse abdominus	Activated in forced exhalation. Strengthening prevents abdominal bulge.	❏	❏	❏
Lower body				
Quadriceps	Worked through both hip and knee movement.	❏	❏	❏
Hamstrings	Hard to isolate without equipment: tight on most participants.	❏	❏	❏
Gastrocnemius	Worked mostly with a straight leg.	❏	❏	❏
Soleus	Worked mostly with a bent leg.	❏	❏	❏
Tibialis anterior	Very weak muscle, which can be easily overloaded in impact activities; may require strengthening.	❏	❏	❏
Adductors	Hard to isolate, especially without equipment.	❏	❏	❏
Abductors	Often given more emphasis than they deserve.	❏	❏	❏

KEY:
L–Light workout; M–Moderate workout; I–Intense workout.

Table 9.1. **Evaluation of muscle balance**

Muscle balance

Muscle imbalance can easily be created outside of the fitness centre through various lifestyle factors, such as posture, occupation, activity or lack of activity. A well-designed progressive resistance training program can help restore and maintain proper muscle balance.

All muscles or groups of muscles work in pairs—the agonist and antagonist. When one of the muscles is actively shortened, the other is passively stretched. Thus, if one muscle group becomes disproportionately stronger than the other, it can exert stretching forces that can be greater than the weaker muscle can withstand, and an injury can occur from this imbalance. For instance, excessive quadriceps strength and a weaker hamstring can cause such injuries as a 'pulled hamstring'. All muscle groups can be affected by this imbalance, and one of the results causing great concern is an undesirable change in posture.

When evaluating or planning a muscle-conditioning routine you can check muscle balance using Table 9.1 as a guide. Place a tick inside the box indicating how much that muscle has been worked in a whole class or single routine in class.

Major positional exercises

Position	Basic exercise	Common variations
Standing	Lunge	Forwards, backwards
	Squat	Wide, mid-stance, narrow
Prone	Push-ups	Wide, narrow, staggered, on knees or extended
	Abdominals	Lying flat pelvic set, on knees, on toes
	Opposite arm-leg	Single arm or leg extension
	Back extensions	Different arm position
Supine	Crunch	Full, staggered, rotation
	Reverse crunch	Heels close to gluteals, legs extended to ceiling
	Lateral flexion	Short reach, long reach
	Dips	Legs extended, heels close to pelvis
Side lying	Oblique crunch	With rotation

Table 9.2. **Basic non-equipment exercises in the four primary body positions**

Effective cueing for muscle conditioning

As the music used in muscle conditioning is of a slower speed, and little travel is involved, the instructor is able to provide a high level of cueing. Particular attention should be given to technical cueing. The most common form of cueing involves the four stages of What, Where, When and How (see Chapter 4). The What refers to the name or the common exercise vocabulary; the Where refers to direction of travel, e.g. lunge fwd; the When is your countdown or preparatory stage; and the How refers to the technical description. Following the technical description, imagery is used to ensure your participants have a sound understanding of the movements being executed, and this can also be used to lift the level of performance or commitment to the exercise.

When making corrections, ensure that you talk to the whole group. Specific eye contact can be directed at those individuals who need additional correction and you may even need to go to the person and make physical adjustments to their technique or position. Remember to touch hard points only, and try first to get alongside the participant so they can mirror your position.

Continually change your position of demonstration to ensure that all participants have a clear view of your body position. The following stages are an easy-to-follow guide when instructing:
1. Cue position relative to anatomy.
2. Emphasise the effort phase.
3. Use sensory or imagery cues.

Table 9.3 outlines some technical cues and associated imagery for basic non-equipment muscle-conditioning exercises. You may develop your own cues for imagery that work best for your centre or country.

Basic exercise	Technical cue	Imagery
Standing (see Fig. 9.1)		
Lunge	Hips and shoulders square, legs 2 x shoulder width long, 1 x shoulder width wide. Distribute weight evenly between legs, knees over mid-foot.	Keep knees soft, point hips forward to the front, sink down, trunk vertical.
Squat	Keep knees in line with the mid-foot. Weight evenly distributed between feet. Hips pushed backwards. Avoid locking the knees.	Toes peeping out under knees. Feet turned out at 10 and 2 o'clock. Sit down on a chair.
Prone (see Fig. 9.2)		
Push-ups	Keep shoulders relaxed, elbows bend first. Modify to the knees for beginners, hands under shoulders.	Tighten abdominals, back straight. Keep shoulders out of ears, and elbows soft at all times.
Abdominals		
Level 1 (L1)–pelvic set. Lie on stomach with shoulders & elbows on the floor	L1–Set the pelvis in a neutral position, breathe in, then narrow the waist as you breathe out. Tighten the abdominals and hold for 16 counts then release	L1–Take a big deep breath in and breathe out to shrink the waist and tighten the area. Imagine you are wearing a corset.
Level 2 (L2)–pelvic lift. Lift upper body up onto the elbows	L2–Maintain set position as you draw pelvis/hips off the ground. Maintain neutral spinal alignment, hold for 16–32 counts and release.	
Level 3 (L3)–knee lift. Start on elbows, with pelvis lifted off floor.	L3–Maintain set position then lift knees so that body is lifted onto the toes. Hold position to fatigue, then lower onto knees.	
Opposite arm-leg extension	Place hands in front and look at the ground, lift opposite arm and leg simultaneously. Hold at the top, lower and repeat other side.	Lengthen the body. Draw the arm and leg to the ceiling. Focus on the long muscles that run along the spine. Eyes stay low and relax the neck.
Lower back extension	Place backs of fingers on forehead, elbows are bent and resting on floor. Legs and hips are flat on the floor. Slowly raise the trunk off the ground. Look at the ground and relax the neck. Hold at the top and slowly lower upper body to start position.	Feel your hips and toes on the ground. Upper body should be straight and strong as you lift.
Supine (see Fig. 9.3)		
Crunch	Keep head in line with spine. Flex the trunk approx. 30–45° so that the shoulders lift up. Use your hands to support your head, or alternatively lay hands on thighs or cross at chest.	Keep the chin off the chest to leave enough space under your chin to fit a tennis ball or piece of fruit. Bring the ribs towards the hips.
Reverse crunch	Lift hips to clear floor. Avoid swinging legs and use hands to support under the hips if needed.	Keep ankles close to the gluteals and move hips to the ribs.
Dips	Ensure elbows are first to bend. Keep shoulders depressed. If using a bench, keep the buttocks close so that the back is vertical.	Keep shoulders out of ears. Close your armpits. Keep elbows soft.
Side Lying (see Fig. 9.4)		
Oblique crunch	Lift shoulders off floor and take ribs towards hips. Place lower arm on floor if support is needed.	Reach your shoulder towards your knees. Knees are stuck to the floor.

Table 9.3. **Technical cues and imagery for basic non-equipment muscle-conditioning exercises**

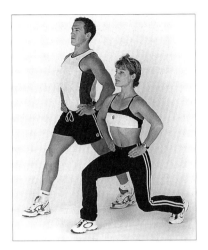

1. Lunge

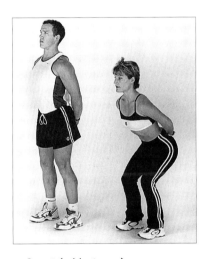

2. Squat (mid-stance)

Fig. 9.1. Standing exercises

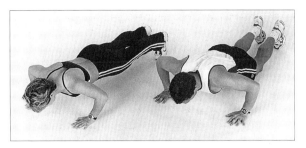

1. Push-ups (on toes, on knees)

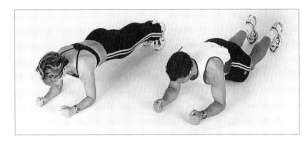

2. Prone abdominals (Levels 2 and 3)

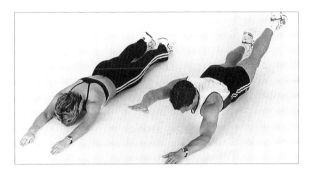

3. Opposite arm-leg extension

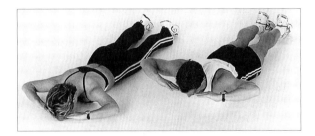

4. Lower back extension

Fig. 9.2. Prone exercises

principles of muscle conditioning

Getting results — Key principles of muscle conditioning

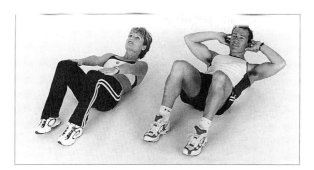

1. Crunch (hands on thighs, hands supporting head)

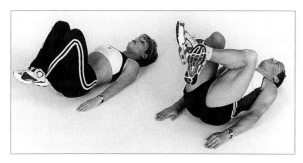

2. Reverse crunch

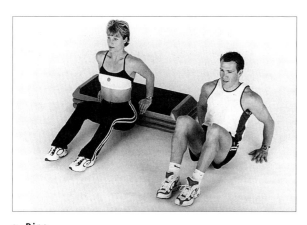

3. Dips

Fig. 9.3. Supine exercises

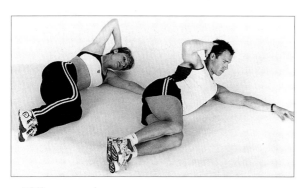

1. Oblique crunch

Fig. 9.4. Side-lying exercise

Overload is the key to improvement in any form of muscle conditioning or resistance training. Overload refers to loading a muscle to the point where changes have to occur in the motor units, both structurally and chemically, in order for the muscle to adapt to a new load. There are many ways to achieve overload during exercise. These include increasing the repetitions, increasing the weight used, and reducing recovery time. Keeping the intensity level high may be as simple as changing your rest time from 1 minute to approximately 30 seconds. Involvement in new activities and exercises, along with thoughtful sequencing of exercises, will all assist in creating overload.

The principles of overload can be adapted into any muscle-conditioning class format to assist you in creating a varied, quality workout for your participants. A variety of techniques is listed below. Examples include both body weight and hand weights.

Pyramiding/reverse pyramiding

Repetitions are either increased or decreased. Common combinations can be 1, 2, 4, 8 and then reversing the number of repetitions. This technique can be performed with either a single exercise or a combination of exercises.

Practical application of pyramiding

| Move A | Wide squat |
| Move B | Narrow squat |

Start with 1 repetition (rep.) of each move, then increase to 2, 4 and 8 reps of each move.

Negative reps

Eccentric contractions are commonly referred to as a negative rep. By emphasising the eccentric contraction, participants can learn to improve their coordination and control of movement. Training muscles eccentrically can be a useful technique in injury prevention. An emphasis on eccentric contractions can be achieved in class through the use of rhythm.

Practical application of negative reps

Wide squat	Down 1–3, up on 4
(Toes at 10 and 2 o'clock)	Down 1–7, up on 8
	Down 1-15, up on 16

Range of movement (ROM) method

Often referred to as 'Matrix training', this technique involves manipulating the ROM of each exercise. The full ROM is divided into two halves, i.e. the upper and lower ranges. The first half of the motion is performed (upper or lower) and then the second half of the motion is performed. To conclude this set, the full range of motion is then performed.

When using this method in class, the half-range movements need to be performed at normal time and the full range needs to be performed at half time (slower). The most common repetition sequences are 4–4–8 or 8–8–16.

Practical application of ROM method

Move	ROM
Dips x 4	Ground to halfway up
Dips x 4	Halfway to full extension
Dips x 4	Full ROM

Super Sets

There are two main types of Super Set techniques. The first is outlined below under 'Push Pull' method and the second involves programming several exercises for the same muscle group or body part in succession (also known as 'Compound Setting'). Generally three exercises are sequenced together for the one muscle group or body part.

Practical application of Super Set/Compound Set
Shoulders using dumbbells

Exercise 1	Lateral raise
Exercise 2	Overhead press
Exercise 3	Upright row

The Push Pull involves performing an exercise for the agonist followed by an exercise for the antagonist muscle.

Practical application of Super Set/Push Pull
Arms using dumbbells

Move A	Hammer curls (biceps)
Move B	Tricep kickback (triceps)

Pre-exhaustion

A technique where a muscle is worked firstly in isolation and then followed by working the muscle in a compound exercise. In the isolation exercise, the muscle is worked to the point of 'exhaustion' but can continue to work in the compound exercise due to the involvement of the other prime movers. In class, this method can be achieved by using a single-joint then a multi-joint action.

Practical application of pre-exhaustion
Triceps pre-exhaustion using a barbell (supine on a bench)

Exercise 1	Triceps press
Exercise 2	Chest press

Ensure that you have a thorough understanding of each muscle and its function before applying muscle conditioning to your classes. A variety of well-planned muscle-conditioning routines can create a safe and effective phase to any class. Whether incorporated into a complete class format or a phase of a class, muscle conditioning can benefit participants in preventing injury, improving body composition, providing muscular balance and improving strength and endurance.

Equipment-Based Muscle Conditioning

While body weight can provide adequate overload for many exercises such as push-ups, crunches and lunges, other exercises require extra resistance in order to be effective. Equipment such as hand weights, rubber tubing and resistance bands are discussed in this chapter.

The use of light hand weights

Light weights can create two important factors for aerobics class consideration, including intensity and a 'toning' or conditioning effect for muscles.

Intensity

Energy cost or expenditure can be increased when working with hand weights as opposed to working without them. The major benefits come from increasing the range of movement when working with hand weights rather than trying to increase the tempo of the movements. Obviously, there is a limit to the number of armlines or movements that can be performed, but the options are endless when combining arm and leg patterns in classes.

Toning or conditioning

Most aerobics classes tend to focus on the lower body. By using hand weights, the upper body can be emphasised and create a more balanced, cross training effect. Your participants will be able to notice an increase in muscle definition in their upper body. The Body Sculpt class is specially designed to condition all muscle groups and improve muscular strength and endurance.

Special considerations

Music speed

Each participant will have special needs in terms of their own body shape and size. Music speed for equipment-based muscle conditioning is considerably slower than aerobic music. The speed of music selected will vary according to hand-weight size, lever length (arm length), ROM and stationary vs travelling moves performed. For correct form, technique and full ROM, you will need to instruct participants to keep the weights close to their body at all times when music speed reaches 130–132 bpm. Barbell classes generally focus on strength in a stationary position, and regular Step speed or below is the most suitable music selection. Movements need to be controlled, and for Body Sculpt classes the following music speeds are recommended:

MUSIC	MOVES
70–115 bpm	Strength
120–130 bpm	Stationary
120–132 bpm	Travelling

Exercise selection

Plan to work both small and large muscle groups within your class. Ensure that opposing muscle groups are utilised and that a balanced program is developed for each session. Balancing opposing muscle groups will prevent injuries and assist in maintaining correct posture. Correct exercise sequencing will avoid muscle burnout; the deltoid muscle is one that is particularly susceptible to this condition. Both isolated and compound exercises should be included in each class, with compatible upper and lower body movement patterns to ensure smooth transitions and class flow.

Movements should be performed with the full range of motion, and execution should be smooth. When linking two or more moves, ensure that you consider which muscles are being worked, and the physiological and biomechanical stresses being placed on the muscles and joints. For safety reasons, HIA should never include the use of hand weights. Ankle weights should never be used with LIA or HIA. Do not sacrifice safety in an attempt to increase intensity levels or in a quest for creativity. Alternatives will be made for use with a barbell—these include rhythm variations, ROM and number combinations, which can be incorporated with all the basic exercises.

Lever length

When planning for your classes, you will need to include a good mix of long and short levers and ensure that your music speeds are always within the recommended guidelines. Remember, short arms can always work faster than long arms, so consider your taller and shorter participants. Long lever work may be performed at slower speeds, e.g using rhythm at half time. If the movements are performed at a faster speed or to music that is too fast, momentum may be built. Momentum will increase the risk of injuries to the joints and the muscles.

Always plan and instruct for safety and control. When planning your cueing, power words can be used to help give your participants a clear understanding of what is expected of them. Imagery through these power words and the use of various tones will also assist when instructing. Encourage full ROM when working with the barbell. Movements will generally be slower and more controlled. Power words to assist with lever length can include:

- Place (instead of 'swing');
- Control;
- Squeeze;
- Pull;
- Push;
- Focus.

Participants

Not only will participants have special needs for lever length, but they may also have certain conditions that make using light weights impossible. Participants with such conditions as high blood pressure, RSI, arthritis or joint injuries should avoid this type of exercise.

You may find that two distinct types of participants will be attracted to the muscle conditioning or Body Sculpt class in your centre. These include the 'die hard' enthusiast who essentially wants to overload each muscle group until it is fatigued. This group enjoys a challenge and a great total body workout.

The second type of participant is one who is more concerned with a lighter workout. They want to work all body parts in a class format that resembles a stretch and tone class. This format focuses on control, and participants are encouraged to work at their own pace. Look at your participants' needs and wants. Develop a process for evaluating what type of class format your participants prefer. If you have a good balance of participants, remember to always give suitable levels and 'less fit' variations of each exercise.

Grip

If the weight is gripped too tightly, this may increase peripheral resistance, causing an increase in blood pressure and heart rate. When using any type of light weight or rubberised resistance, a tight grip may also cause and/or aggravate tendon injuries in the forearm or wrist. Allowances should be made for handle and non-handle weights. Ensure that your participants are instructed to use their thumb and a combination of fingers when gripping the weights, barbell or handles. For strength or stationary moves, both hand-held weights can be transferred into one hand to give one arm a rest and overload the other arm. Alternatively, the barbell can be rested on the chest, upper arms or upper back when performing lower body exercises.

Posture

Many different armlines will be used throughout a muscle-conditioning workout. As your participants fatigue or perform armlines that move directly away from the line of the body, e.g. standing tricep press side, they will need constant cues and instructions from you. These cues will remind participants to keep their 'abs tight and chest lifted' to ensure correct body alignment. Participants should be instructed to avoid locking or hyperextending joints. When instructing with a barbell, ensure that both upper body cues and foot placement cues accompany your exercise vocabulary, to ensure correct posture and body alignment. Feet placement may vary between each barbell exercise, depending on individual comfort levels. Power words to assist with posture and technique can include:
- Soft elbows;
- Soft knees;
- Stand tall;
- Tight abs.

Warm-up and cool-down

Ensure that your warm-up directly reflects the type of activity to be performed in your class. The warm-up should be specific to the upper and lower body. You should instruct your participants to warm up and stretch without hand weights and to focus on strong armlines. Some armlines that will be used in the class can be pre-taught in the warm-up to effectively utilise teaching time. The cool-down should focus on increasing flexibility and restoring full range of motion.

Transitional skills

To increase the effectiveness of resistive exercise, ensure that you identify a start and finishing point for each of your moves. Clear cues should be given to participants when you are changing and setting new body positions. Smooth transitions are important. With careful planning and consideration, it will be easy to adjust from one muscle group to another without interrupting the flow of the workout. Quick grip changes can be made when using barbells to eliminate transition time.

Breathing techniques

Specific breathing cues can assist in creating control and body awareness for your participants. You should allow your participants to use their own optimum breathing techniques. Well-educated members will know to exhale on a concentric contraction and inhale on an eccentric contraction, which is the most common form of breathing when performing resistive exercise.

Exercise vocabulary for light hand weights

Listed on the following pages are the common terms or exercise vocabulary used in a Body Sculpt class when using light hand weights. Rhythm variations, ROM and number combinations can be incorporated into the basic exercises when using a barbell. When instructing with a barbell, ensure that cues for upper body, trunk stabilisation and foot placement accompany your exercise vocabulary.

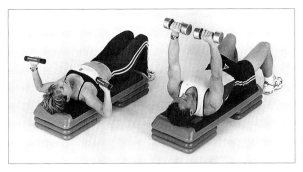
1. Wide chest press

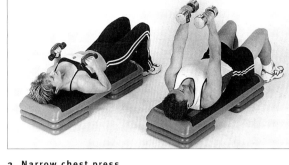
2. Narrow chest press

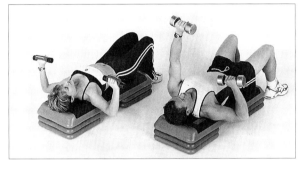
3. Single arm press

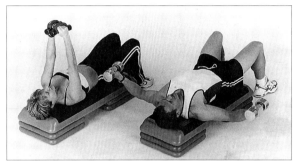
4. Chest fly

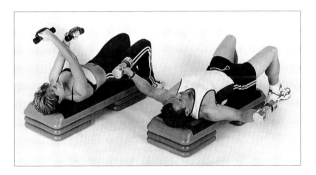
5. Cross fly

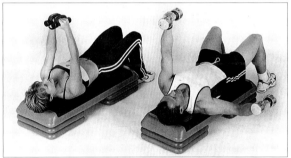
6. Single fly

Fig. 10.1. **Exercises for the chest**

UPPER BODY/CHEST	
Pectorals	Chest press (wide)
	Narrow press
	Single arm press
	Fly
	Cross fly
	Pec-dec

Tip: Pectoral muscles are best worked in a supine position where the 'line of pull' is directly against gravity. By positioning the body on a bench the range of motion is enhanced, therefore increasing effectiveness.

equipment-based muscle conditioning

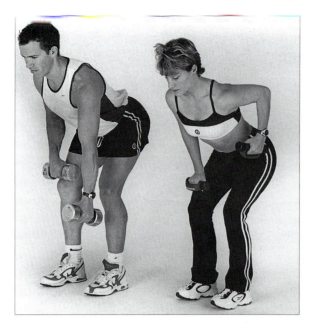

1. Single arm row

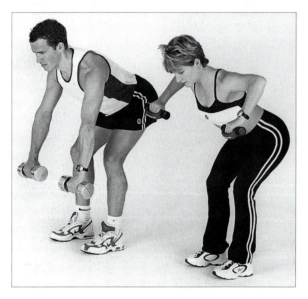

2. Bent over row

Fig. 10.2. **Exercises for the upper and middle back**

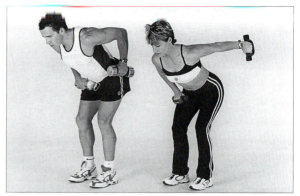

1. Tricep kickback

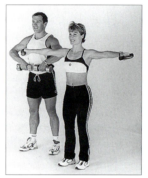

2. Tricep side

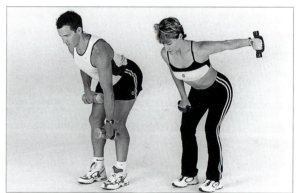

3. Tricep lift back

Fig. 10.3. **Exercises for the triceps**

UPPER AND MIDDLE BACK	
Rhomboids/Mid trapezius/	Bent-over row
Posterior deltoid	Reverse fly
Lats	Single arm row
	Bent-over row
Tip: Supported forward flexion held for short periods is considered acceptable for these exercises. Ensure good body alignment is performed.	

ARM	
Triceps	Tricep kickback (extension)
	Tricep side (extend to side)
	Lift back (elbows extended)
Tip: In elbow extension, keep the elbow in a horizontal line with the shoulder. Avoid locking the elbow.	

the aerobics instructor's handbook

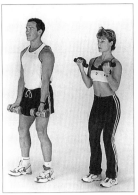 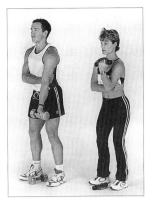 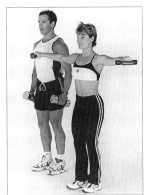 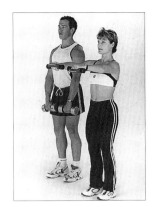

1. Bicep curl   2. Bicep preacher curl   1. Lateral raise (long lever)   2. Front raise

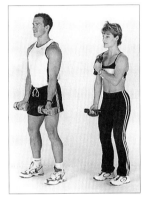 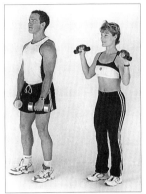 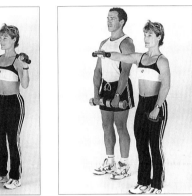 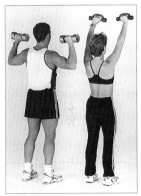

3. Across the body curl   4. V-hammer curl   3. Alt. front raise   4. Shoulder press

Fig. 10.4. **Exercises for the biceps**

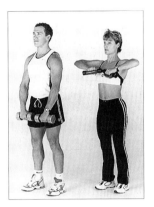 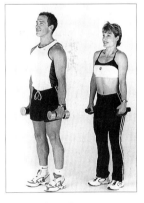

5. Upright row   6. Shoulder shrug

Fig. 10.5. **Exercises for the shoulder**

ARM	
Biceps	Bicep curl
	Side curl
	Preacher curl
	Across the body curl
	V-hammer curl

Tip: When flexing the elbow, keep the armpit closed and perform with control. Avoid locking the elbow on lowering the weight.

SHOULDER	
Deltoid	Lateral raise (short/long lever)
	Front raise
Trapezius	Shoulder press
	Upright row
	Shoulder shrug

Tip: Avoid the 'deltoid burnout' produced through too many shoulder exercises or repetitions.

equipment-based muscle conditioning

The use of rubberised resistance

The use of rubberised resistance (RR) equipment is a well established alternative for muscle conditioning. RR is a variable form of resistance, where greater resistance is experienced as the rubber is stretched. RR includes fit strips or resistance bands and tubes with handles. RR allows instructors to work muscles in a range of positions and it is an effective means of developing muscular strength. Strip bands can be used, either tied or untied for variety and additional resistance.

Special considerations

When introducing new equipment in your class, ensure that you outline the following safety considerations:
- Pre-class screening must be performed to identify any joint injuries, and conditions such as high blood pressure and arthritis. These are the main contraindications when working with RR.
- Have all participants scan their bands or tubing for any cuts, tears or weak points either at the handles or throughout the band.
- Check your aerobics area and participant numbers to ensure there is safety and adequate space for participants to perform their required movements.
- Continually cue and educate your participants on correct breathing techniques. Remind them not to hold their breath at any stage during the exercise or workout; encourage rhythmic breathing.

Teaching tips

Overload is easily achieved, so exercises should be selected to alternate muscle groups and avoid burnout. As discussed previously, the deltoid muscle is one that fatigues quickly. To avoid this fatigue and overuse, alternate muscle groups or use one arm at a time, or alternate exercises for the lower body and upper body. You should always start slowly with low reps and try not to confuse participants by adding too many exercises into the one workout.

Quality always wins over quantity, so emphasise technique, form and correct alignment. Each side of the body should be worked evenly, with intensity and number of reps staying constant. Avoid overusing the first side and rushing to finish the second side. Make certain that equal time is given to each muscle group.

Music speed

Music speeds for RR should remain around 115–120 bpm to ensure a slow and controlled movement.

Teaching techniques

- There should be an absence of jerky, uncontrolled movements associated with letting the band go 'slack'. The resistance needs to remain constant throughout each exercise.
- Always allow time at the start of the class and at the start of a new muscle-conditioning phase of the class to explain the correct placement of hands and feet with the bands or tubing.
- The wrist should always remain an extension of the arm. Avoid wrist hyperextension and hyperflexion; keep it firm and in a neutral position.
- Participants should always be in control of their movements. Don't let the band control you.
- Always keep joints relaxed and soft. Avoid squeezing the handles or gripping the band too tightly. This tends to elevate the blood pressure or falsely increase the heart rate.
- Intensity can be increased by shortening the band.

Continually repeat your body checks throughout the workout. Tips for correct posture include: 'Stand tall, abdominals tight, head up, shoulders back and down, knees relaxed and slightly bent, the back should be straight and relaxed'.

Drill

Design a comprehensive muscle conditioning workout for the upper body combination, using RR. Consider starting points, flow, transitions and deltoid burnout.

Muscle-conditioning classes

There are various alternative formats for muscle conditioning classes. Table 10.1 provides three suggestions.

Format A	Format B	Format C
Warm-up	Warm-up	Warm-up
LIA (optional)	LIA (optional)	LIA (optional)
Standing upper body work	Standing upper body work	Hand weight/barbell resistive work OR
Supported/floor upper body work	Standing leg work	Rubberised band resistive work AND
Standing leg work	Floor/bench upper body work	Step supported resistive work
Supported/floor leg work	Floor leg work	
Abdominal	Abdominals	Abdominals
Lower back	Lower back	Lower back
Cool-down	Cool-down	Cool-down

Table 10.1. **Alternative formats for muscle-conditioning classes**

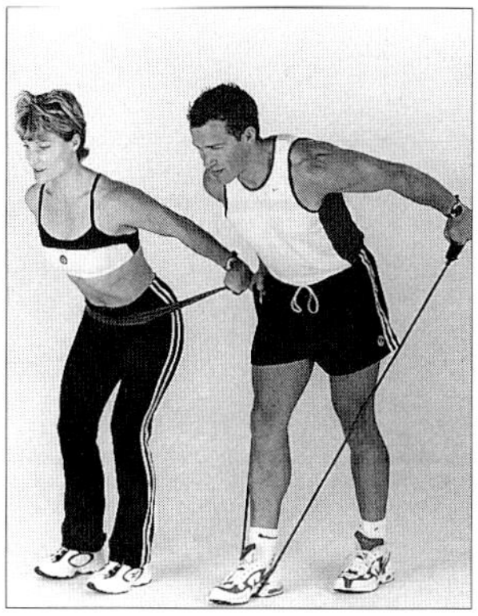

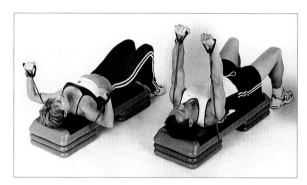

Fig. 10.7 **Tricep kickback**

Tricep kickback: Step on RR with one or both feet; knees should be slightly bent. With palms facing body, grasp handles or ends. Elbows remain elevated and close to your sides. Push both or one arm backwards and extend at the elbows. Alternatively, place a band around the hips and perform a sgl or dbl tricep kickback.

Exercise vocabulary for tubing and fit strips

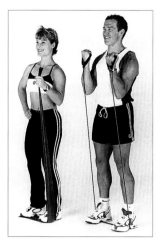

Fig. 10.6. **Bicep curl**

Bicep curl: Step on RR with one or both feet; knees should be slightly bent with palms facing body; grasp handles or ends. Elbows should be close to the body as both hands are lifted towards the shoulders then lowered.

Fig. 10.8. **Chest press**

Chest press: Lie flat on the platform with feet together on the ground close to end of step. Knees are bent to support the back. The RR is placed under the platform and held beside the chest with each hand, knuckles to the roof. Arms slowly rise together straight up until arms are extended. Elbows should remain slightly bent and the wrist will be in line with the forearm. Slowly lower to start.

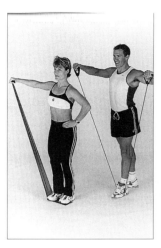

Fig. 10.9. **Lateral raise**

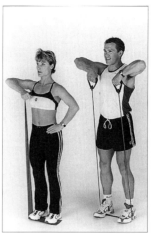

Fig. 10.11. **Upright row**

Lateral raise: Step on RR with one or both feet; knees should be slightly bent. Arms are held away from body to the side of the thighs, with little or no tension on the RR. Move arms away from your sides until the wrist lines up with the shoulders. Slowly lower to start. Keep elbows soft. If participants are tall, offer a single lateral raise which will be easier to achieve.

Upright row: Step on RR with one or both feet; knees should be slightly bent. Arms are held in front of the body at thigh level. Palms are facing inwards, elbows remain slightly bent and the wrist in line with the forearm. Pull up slowly with either one or both arms, raising elbows to shoulder level.

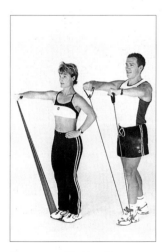

Fig. 10.10. **Front raise**

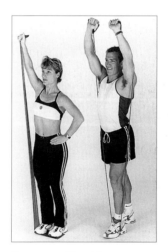

Fig. 10.12. **Shoulder press**

Front raise: Step on RR with one or both feet; knees should be slightly bent. Arms are held in front of the body at the thighs. Arms are raised together, or one at a time, straight in front against the tension. Elbows should remain slightly bent and the wrist will be in line with the forearm.

Shoulder press: Step on RR with one or both feet; knees should be slightly bent. Hands are at shoulder level. Start by extending one or two arms overhead. This will depend on the participant's height and the length of the RR. Tall individuals should perform a single shoulder press, then change arms. Wrist remains in line with the forearm.

the aerobics instructor's handbook

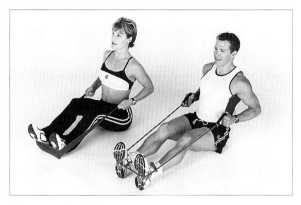

Fig. 10.13. **Seated row**

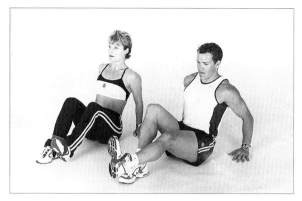

Fig. 10.15. **Leg press**

Seated row: Start in a seated position, keeping knees soft and toes pointed slightly forward throughout. Link the band around the feet and bring hands at or just above waist level. Pull back and end with elbows behind the body. Palms remain facing in to body and close to sides at all times.

Leg press: Tie the RR at the ends to form a circular band. The band is placed round the ankle of the stabilising or support leg and around the foot of the working leg. Push the foot forward, straightening the leg against the resistance.

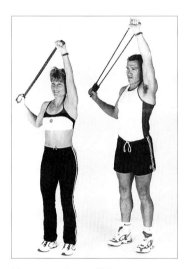

Fig. 10.14. **Lat pulldown**

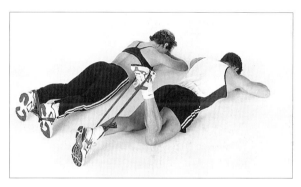

Fig. 10.16. **Leg curl**

Lat pulldown: Arms are placed overhead in the starting position. Keep one arm stable and firm and pull the other arm down. The wrist remains in line with the forearm. Return to starting position.

Leg curl: Tie the RR at the ends to form a circular band. Lie flat on your stomach, chest on floor. The band is placed around the ankle of the stabilising or support leg and around the foot of the working leg. Slowly bend at the knee and bring the foot towards the buttocks. Head can rest on upper arms.

Step Classes

First used for fitness testing and rehabilitation programs, Step has developed into one of the most widely known forms of aerobics. Walking up and down stairs is such a common part of everyday life, and had never been considered a structured exercise program until the late '80s–early '90s. Its popularity has continued to increase due to its athletic nature, simplicity, and the research behind the Step program. Another asset to the program has been the instructor skill development and commitment. Step is a fun workout with easy-to-follow moves that produce great results.

The strengths of Step

Today, Step Aerobics is widely enjoyed in the aerobics studio and in the pool because its moves are simple and easy to learn. It provides a great cardiovascular and strengthening workout, as the platform can be used for many different functions besides basic stepping. It only requires slightly more space per participant than a standard aerobics class. Step energy expenditure is equivalent to walking at 6.5 km (4 miles) per hour up to jogging at approximately 8–11 km (5–7 miles) per hour, with intensity varying with each participant. The exact energy costs will depend on step height, speed of music, individual body weight and gender.

Stepping safely

The following teaching guidelines must be incorporated into your instructions to participants in Step classes. They can be included in an INTRO or your general class cueing system.

- Ensure that the whole foot is placed on the step throughout the class. Ask participants to check that their heels are not hanging over the back of the step, especially towards the end of the workout when fatigue may have set in. Achilles tendonitis and calf soreness can occur due to incorrect heel and foot placement. Newcomers may need to look down to check their step quite regularly if they are unsure about their feet placement and step technique.

- Stand close to the step. Avoid stepping too far from the back of the step. This will interrupt your participants' step pattern and timing and can also cause Achilles and calf soreness.
- Step softly onto the step and cue the correct foot placement. The heel should contact the step platform first. The cues should include 'roll through the foot and contact heel–toe'. This will enable the toe to clear the front of the step also. When stepping down from the platform the cues should include 'roll down from toe to heel'. This will allow for maximum absorption of impact and an overall reduction in the impact forces.
- Set up platforms with adequate space around and between each one. This will ensure that participants won't step on other platforms or fellow participants.
- Balance the use of lead legs. Ensure that both right and left leg leads are performed throughout each class and each combination. You cannot rely on your finished product to provide the only lead leg balance when the teaching progressions do not reflect this. The introduction of Step has made us aware of the importance of maintaining equal balance between left and right lead legs. One leg should lead continually for a maximum of 1 minute before changing to the opposite leg.
- Cue your participants to 'stand tall, hold abdominals tight, shoulders back, head and neck relaxed and up'. Continually observe and correct posture and knee alignment. Avoid instructing with too much forward flexion on rear lift moves.
- Any additional equipment should be placed underneath the step and out of the way of foot placement.
- No hand weights should be used when combining complex leg patterns or when performing 'propulsions' or power moves in Step. Leg patterns should be simple to complement the use of hand weights and strong armlines.
- Vary armlines when stepping to avoid the overuse of the shoulder joint.
- If armlines interfere with leg patterns, participants should be instructed to keep the arms by their side, on hips or hold with a natural swing or running action. The leg patterns and the use of large muscle groups are the most important factor to ensure that participants benefit from the cardiovascular workout of Step.
- Participants should be educated on correct step height. The knee joint should not bend more than 90 degrees.
- Step height can be reduced or increased during the class to increase or decrease intensity levels.
- Follow the Step music guidelines to ensure safe stepping at all times. This is your responsibility as a professional.
- Follow the guidelines set for you by your fitness centre in relation to class description and content.
- Step is suitable for all fitness and ability levels. However, attempt to screen all participants before they commence the Step program. Participants with chronic back or joint problems, pregnant women, newcomers, over-40s, and individuals with high blood pressure should seek permission from their physicians before commencing a Step program. Ensure that newcomers start with a Step introduction class to learn all the rules.

The wrong steps

Stepping up backwards

Stepping up onto the platform with the back facing the step ('stepping blind') makes it virtually impossible for exercisers to be totally aware of their foot placement and the distance of the step from their feet. This type of stepping should be avoided at all times to ensure that your participants do not trip or fall.

Turning movements with loaded knee joints

When you are standing on one leg, the knee is considered loaded. A loaded joint is one that is bearing weight. Injury can potentially occur when attempting turning movements when the knee is loaded. When turning, always lift the heel and unload the leg to transfer the weight onto the ball of the foot. This will allow the foot to turn easily on the step. No pivoting movements should be performed when the body weight is supported through the knee.

Stepping down forwards

Even though we walk forwards down stairs in everyday life, repeated forward stepping can increase the risk of knee injuries. Stepping down forwards off the step should be avoided.

Jumping off the step

Plyometric training of athletes involves propulsions or jumping actions from steps or heights. This training is suitable for elite athletes, but not your regular participants. A high risk of injury exists for the feet, knees and lower back areas. You should not instruct your participants to jump from the top of the step to the floor.

Crossing the feet when stepping

When travelling over or across the top of the step, the feet should not be crossed. It will increase the risk of participants tripping when travelling over the step.

Step heights

The following are recommended step heights for your participants, based on their experience, fitness level and body height:

10 cm step platform (4 inches). Suitable for deconditioned or beginner participants who have not exercised for some time, or a shorter, conditioned participant.
20 cm step platform (8 inches). Suitable for a conditioned participant who exercises regularly. Suitable for an average height or taller conditioned participant.
30 cm step platform (12 inches). Suitable for medium to advanced regular participants or taller exercisers. *Note:* Platform only (no risers) is recommended for deconditioned, elderly and pregnant participants.

Step music speeds

The recommended music speed for Step is 118–124 bpm. More experienced participants can successfully step at speeds up to 128 bpm, but this should only be used in advanced classes. Most Step classes have mixed ability levels where slower speeds are more suitable. All classes should commence with lower speeds for the first few music tracks. Until your participants' ability level improves, the lower range is more suitable for accurate alignment, full range of motion and control of movements. Remember, an increase in music speed does not necessarily mean an increase in intensity or motivation.

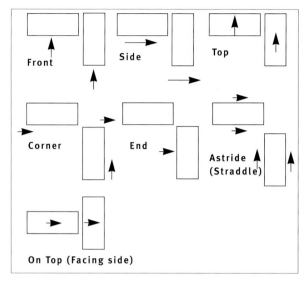

Fig. 11.1. **Starting positions**

The base moves and Step vocabulary

As in aerobics, there are only a few categories of base Step moves (e.g. basic, lift steps, tap steps) from which numerous variations are formed. The most common Step moves and variations follow. The 'lead leg' refers to the first foot placed on the step. The 'trail leg' is the other foot, which is placed on the step to complete the move.

Basic step up/down

Description: A basic step is the most common foot pattern of Step moves. The move is executed for a right leg lead by R foot up, L foot up, R foot down, L foot down. A left foot lead basic step is executed by L foot up, R foot up, L foot down, R foot down. It is very similar to marching, where the legs keep the same pattern R, L, R, L, etc.
Special considerations: The whole foot of both the lead and trail leg is placed on the step. Ensure power moves are done onto the step and not onto the floor.

Knees will be slightly flexed when stepping up and down.
Variations or examples: Single or alternate lead leg, basic step down, power leap up (one foot lead), power jump up (both feet lead), basic step up with 2 alternating lunges from on top of the step and basic down (8-count move).
Starting position: Front, end, or astride or top for basic step down.
Common cueing: Up, up, down, down (4-count move).

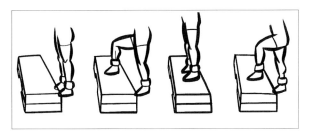

Fig. 11.2. Basic step

V-step

Description: The V-step is performed to form a V-shape on the step and the floor. The right foot steps up and out, the L foot steps up and out, the R foot steps down and centre and the L foot steps down and centre.
Special considerations: Ensure legs are placed back together in the centre and not wide on the down phase of the step. Keep the whole foot of both the lead and trail leg on the step. The feet will be slightly turned out when placed up on the step to compensate for knee angles and for safety.
Variations or examples: Single or alternate lead leg.
Starting position: Front.
Common cueing: Wide, wide, down, down *or* out, out, in, in (4-count moves).

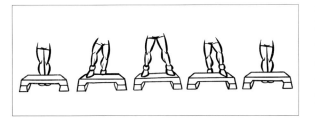

Fig. 11.3. **V-step**

Lift steps

Description: The lift step is an alternating step which changes the lead leg each time the move is performed. It involves the lead leg stepping onto the step and the trail leg lifts. The lifted leg is then lowered to the ground followed by the leg on the step. For example, the footwork for a knee up would be R foot up, L knee lift, L foot down, R foot down, L foot up, R knee lift, R foot down, L foot down.
Special considerations: Ensure that the whole foot of the lead leg is placed on the step.
Variations or examples: Single or alternate lead leg, knee lift, abductor (side) lift, gluteal squeeze (rear), hamstring curl, front kick, combined with straddle (4-count moves).
Starting position: Front, side, end or astride.
Common cueing: Single lift—up, lift, down, tap *or* alternate lift—up, lift, down, down.

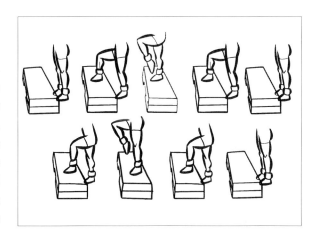

Fig. 11.4. **Lift step (knee) leading right leg then left leg**

Repeater lift (3 continuous lifts)

Description: The repeater is an alternating step where the non–weight-bearing phase of the movement is repeated. A repeater knee lift is performed by R foot up, L knee lift (1), L foot tap down, L knee lift (2), L foot tap down, L knee lift (3), L foot step down, R foot step down. With a left leg lead; L foot up, R knee lift (1), R foot tap down, R knee lift (2), R foot tap down, R knee lift (3), R foot step down, L foot down.
Special considerations: To reduce the amount of stress experienced by the support leg, do not perform

more than 5 repeaters per side at a time. This can be done by performing an 8-count repeater and by applying a variety of lift moves. Touch the floor gently when repeating the action with the trail leg.

Variations or examples: L-step, Rocking horse or T-step, 3 alternating knees or leg curls on top of step (off each side of step = 8 counts); 5 touch repeaters are a variation to the 3 touch repeater move. The 5 touch repeater creates a 12-count move and an additional 4-count move can be added to create a 16-count move combination.

Starting position: Front, side, end or astride.

Common cueing: Repeater—Step, lift, tap, lift, tap, lift, down, down (8 counts).

Turn step

Description: The turn step can be described as an alternating step with a 180 degree turn or a turning alternating V-step. It is generally done from the back of the step and facing the centre. The majority of the platform is used during the execution of this move, or a smaller turn step can also be performed. Execution of the turn step involves: R foot up and quarter turn to the front, L foot up, R foot down and quarter turn to face the centre, L foot tap down. And for a left leg lead: L foot up and a quarter turn to front, R foot up, L foot down and quarter turn to face centre, R foot tap down.

Special considerations: Ensure that the turn is performed on the step while the foot is non–weight-bearing, rather than trying to turn the grounded foot on the floor. Foot placement and correct body positioning in relation to the step are essential to execute the turn step safely. Ensure that the body is facing the centre and that all moves preceding the turn step allow for a safe transition.

Variations or examples: Single or alternate lead leg (continual turns = 4-count moves).

Combinations: Around the world, where a turn step and OTT are combined; single combined with a straddle move (U-turn) cued as 'turn, straddle, turn' (8 - count moves).

Starting position: Front, side or end.

Common cueing: Up, turn, down, tap or turn, turn, down, tap.

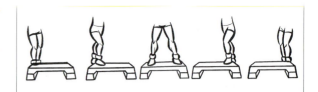

Fig. 11.5. Turn step

Over the top (OTT)

Description: Over the top involves stepping over the top of the step platform. R foot up, L foot up, R foot down on R side of the platform, L foot tap down on R side of the platform, L foot up, R foot up, L foot down on the L side of platform, R foot tap down on L side of platform.

Variations or examples: A-step, switch curl (leg curl switches behind lead leg when moving OTT), corner to corner (4-count moves).

Starting position: Side.

Common cueing: Up, over, down, tap.

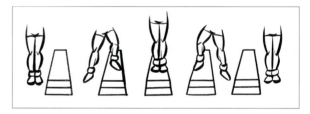

Fig. 11.6. OTT

Across the top (ATT)

Description: Travelling from one end of the step across to the other end of the step. R foot up, L foot up, R foot down on R end of the platform, L foot tap down on R end of platform, L foot up, R foot up, L foot down on the L end of platform, R foot tap down on L end of platform.

Special considerations: A propulsion may be required to assist participants in travelling ATT. This may be common for shorter participants. Offer a low impact version to participants, such as heel or toe tap on each end or a double step touch on the floor.

Variations or examples: Heel or toe tap on top (4-count moves).

Starting position: End.

Common cueing: Up, up, down, tap, or across, down, tap.

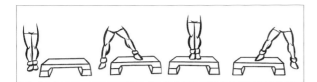

Fig. 11.7. ATT

Lunge steps

Description: The lunge step is a touch pattern that alternates lead legs. From on top: R foot tap down, R foot on top, L foot tap down, left foot on top.

Special considerations: Lunges should be taught at a slower tempo before increasing the speed or adding a propulsion. The heel of the lunging leg should not make contact with the floor unless the lunges are slow. The lunging leg should be lowered onto the ball of the foot first. Lunges should be executed close to the step, to avoid lower leg injury or spinal misalignment. Armlines should be complimentary or rested on the thighs for support during the lunge. The 1-minute time limit should be considered when performing consecutive lunges.

Variations or examples: Single single double, fours, squats, lateral and behind.

Starting position: Top.

Common cueing: Tap down right, on top right, tap down left, on top left.

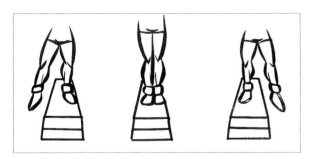

Fig. 11.8. **Lunge step**

Straddle

Description: The straddle can be executed by stepping down from the top of the platform to astride (i.e. one leg either side of the platform) or by stepping from astride to on top of the platform. Straddle down includes; R foot down on R side of the platform, L foot down on L side of the platform into the straddle position, then step R foot up, L foot up. The straddle up involves R foot up, L foot up, R foot down, L foot down.

Special considerations: Ensure the foot placement is wide enough to straddle the platform and keep knees soft. Watch foot placement to avoid tripping on the platform on the way up or down.

Variations or examples: Single or alternating (4-count moves), indecision straddle (8-count move starting from side-on—up, up, straddle, down, up, up, down, tap).

Starting position: Top or side.

Common cueing: Down, down, up, up, or straddle down, up, up.

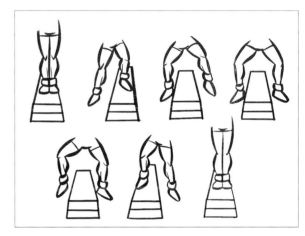

Fig. 11.9. **Straddle down/up**

Tap step

Description: The tap step is a double change pattern and is executed R foot up, L foot tap, L foot down, R foot tap.

Special considerations: The tap is not a weight bearing move. Ensure that the foot lightly taps the floor or the step platform.

Variations or examples: Single or alternating, cha, cha, cha (on top), power jump (on top), mambo (4-count moves), repeater tap up, repeater march stomp (8-count moves).

Starting position: Front, top, astride, end, or corner

Common cueing: Up, tap, down, tap, or the reverse: down, tap, up, tap.

Step choreography and teaching trends

Basic stepping

This involves the basic step moves and a strong emphasis on easy-to-follow patterns. An equal amount of time is spent on and off the step, with little directional variation.

'On the top' mixes

When performing a series of 'on the top' mixes, the moves and the emphasis of movement sequences will have participants remaining on the top of the step for an extended time. Rhythm changes can be performed with basic steps to get participants from the floor to a position on top of the step to perform floor mixes, e.g. half time slow step up R (1, 2), up L (3, 4), step down R (5), down L (6), up R (7), up L (8) where the step sequence finishes on top of the step.

To get from the top of the step to the floor, again rhythm can be used or a series of repeater moves, e.g. from the top of the step, the right leg can perform a touch repeater, such as tap down R (1), up (2), tap down R (3), up (4), tap down (5), up (6), step down R (7), down L (8) to finish on the floor.

Other variations or examples from moves performed on top of the step include: squat, touch steps, step touch, lunges, lift moves, e.g. knee, side, curl, rear, etc.

Floor mix steps

Each of the basic steps moves can be combined with a basic aerobic move, either LIA or HIA. The emphasis will be on activity performed on the floor. HIA moves will be down on the floor rather than on top of the step, for safety.

Variations or examples include: marching (4 or 8 counts) around step or in place, easy walk, star jumps, mambo (on or off the step), step touch, grapevines, squat press, heel digs, squats, etc. The possibilities are endless, providing they are all safe alternatives.

4-, 8-, 16-count transitions

In order to achieve a balance in lead leg, and to move from one side of the step to the other, a transitional move should be performed. This transition can be either 4, 8 or 16 counts and must fit into the choreography sequence. All the examples below change the lead leg.

Examples of a 4-count transition include: over the top (OTT), across the top (ATT), alternate lift move, corner to corner.

Examples of an 8-count transition combination include: indecision straddle, indecision lunge, OTT with an up, tap, down, tap, turn step with an up, tap, down, tap, or an alternating lift move with a basic step or a repeater.

Examples of the 16-count transition could be an indecision with 3 straddles or 3 squats or 6 alt. lunges, or a 5 knee repeater with a basic step.

Tap-free choreography

This involves teaching a step combination or sequence that allows you to transition from one leg to the other continuously without tapping or interrupting the leg patterns. Sample choreography follows.

TAP-FREE CHOREOGRAPHY				
Counts	Move	Lower Body	Travel	Direction
1–16	A	4 x alt. knee lift R, L	OTS	Face front
1–16	B	4 x basic step R	OTS	Face front
1–16	C	2 x 3 knee repeater	OTS	Face front
1–16	D	4 x alt. leg curls, L, R	OTS	Face front

This combination of 64 counts leads with the right leg but must be repeated with the left leg lead to balance the basic steps. Rather than adding a tap down after the alternating curls to change the lead leg, reduce repetitions as follows to create a 32-count combination that leads right then left. (* transition move.)

Counts	Move	Lower Body	Travel	Direction
1–8	A	2 x alt. knee lift R, L	OTS	Face front
1–8	B	2 x basic step R	OTS	Face front
1–8	C*	1 x 3 knee repeater	OTS	Face front
1–8	D	2 x alt. leg curls L, R	OTS	Face front

Propulsion steps

Propulsion steps, sometimes referred to as 'power moves', are advanced variations of the basic moves. The use of propulsions can greatly enhance the intensity level of the workout. The propulsion makes you lift your body high off the platform in an upwards, controlled manner by forcing the lead leg to push harder off the floor to jump up onto the step or up off the top of the step. Propulsion moves are performed in an upward movement onto the step and are never performed down from the step. Propulsion moves feature an airborne phase and hence should be performed by more experienced Step participants. Sample base moves with an added propulsion could include:

Basic step—basic run, ie. run up, walk or step down (don't jump down).

OTT step—add a leap on top of the step then step down.

Lift step (knee)—add a hop on the supporting leg as the knee lifts, then step down.

Propulsions can be given as an option to your more experienced participants. Ensure that their stepping technique is correct first and educate them to land 'softly' when using propulsions.

Muscle-conditioning ideas with the platform

The step platform can be used to manipulate the body into many different positions for muscle conditioning, as follows:

- A variety of lower body exercises can be performed on top of the step, including squat, calf raise and hip extension. Lower body exercises can also start from on top of the step and the working leg can be placed down onto the floor, e.g. lunges or squats.
- The platform can be used to rest the feet on while performing abdominal exercises to assist in stabilising the lower body.
- The platform can be used when performing push-ups. One hand can be placed on the platform and one on the step, or both hands on the step for variety.
- The platform can be held upright on one end to act as a support for balance to ensure correct body alignment and form. This is ideal for newcomers whose balance and proprioception may not be as good as that of regular participants. Any type of lower body work can be performed in this position, such as lunges or squats.
- Rubberised resistance can also be linked under the platform to create effective band stabilisation and support.
- The platform can be used as a bench to perform chest exercises such as chest press, pullovers and flys.

The more experienced you become at teaching Step, the more you will enjoy the challenge of the different type of combinations or sequences you can create. Continually evaluate your participants' needs and requirements in regard to their intensity and fitness levels. Enjoy the strong athletic workout that the Step class provides and avoid getting carried away with too many choreography challenges. Your participants will love this strong workout.

Class Design and Formats

The following class designs and descriptions can be used at fitness centres throughout the world. Additional names for each class have been listed, as each centre may have their own marketing terms or catchy names for particular classes. These name variations are used specifically for marketing purposes to attract new and existing participants to a new class format, or to educate participants on the content and suitability of each class. These descriptions empower participants in making the choice as to which program they think will best suit their needs. It also sets a standard for instructors to follow, as it outlines the content and format of each class.

Class descriptions

Instructor description & guidelines

Step Introduction
Focus on teaching new participants the basics for Step, including terminology, base moves, step orientation, correct technique and form, and easy-to-follow armlines. Repetitions per move should be kept high.
Suitable for: All fitness and ability levels, especially beginners.
Music speed: 118–124 bpm (lower range more suitable).
Equipment: 10–20 cm (4–8 inches) Step platform, Level 2 maximum height (i.e. the base and 1 block).

Consumer description

Step Introduction
Learn all you need to know for Step, including the terms, the basic steps and the movement patterns at an easy-to-follow pace. The intensity level is up to you. Suitable for all levels, especially new steppers.
Other names: Step Orientation, Step Basics, Step First, Intro Step.

Instructor description & guidelines

Step Athletic
Strong basic armlines and foot patterns. Step height is adjustable and hand weights are optional for upper body conditioning. This is a strong and effective workout for all fitness levels.
Suitable for: All levels, but specific to medium to high fitness levels.
Music speed: 118–126 bpm.
Equipment: 10–30 cm (4–12 inches) step platform, up to Level 4 or 5 (i.e. the base plus 3 to 4 blocks). Hand weights are optional but should not exceed 2 kg. No hand weights with propulsions.

Step Moves
A challenging Step class with the addition of new moves and combinations of a higher skill level.
Suitable for: Medium to high co-ordination levels.
Music speed: 120–128 bpm
Equipment: 10–30cm (4–12 inches) Step platform; hand weights not recommended.

Low Impact
Class contains low impact moves, both travelling and stationary (20–30 mins), followed by muscle conditioning (10–15 mins), then a cool-down. Complexity should be kept to a low to moderate level.
Suitable for: All levels, preferably beginners to medium fitness levels.
Music speed: 136–148 bpm for aerobic phase.
Equipment: No equipment required. Light hand weights may be used in the muscle-conditioning phase.

Hi-Lo
Mixed Impact class with elements of both high and low impact combinations. The extended aerobic phase (20–40 mins) features a variety of combinations and basic moves. This is followed by a muscle conditioning phase (5–15 mins) and cool down.
Suitable for: All fitness levels, as low impact options are offered.
Music speed: 145–165 bpm for aerobic phase.
Equipment: No equipment required. Light hand weights can be used in the muscle-conditioning phase.

Consumer description

Step Athletic
Strong emphasis on easy-to-follow steps and strong armlines make this a simple yet effective workout. Some combinations will be taught and propulsions can be introduced to increase the intensity of the workout.
Other names: Step Power.

Step Moves
Suitable for Step regulars who enjoy the challenge of new combinations and moves. The platform can be adjusted for all fitness levels. No hand weights are used in this workout.
Other names: Advanced Step.

Low Impact
Ideal for new exercisers or those returning to exercise after a short break. This class involves no running or jumping and one foot remains in contact with the floor most of the time. There is a cardiovascular phase followed by muscle conditioning and a great cool-down.
Other names: Low Intensity, Light Pace, Beginners, Low and Light, Gentle Exercise, Nice 'n' Easy

Hi-Lo
A varied workout for those looking to improve or maintain their fitness levels. High and low impact moves are included in this class, with a muscle-conditioning phase.
Other names: Combo Class, Cardio, Total Body.

| Instructor description & guidelines | Consumer description |

High Energy/Impact

This has an extended high energy/impact cardiovascular phase. Combinations consist of simple choreography and basic moves, both travelling and stationary. Organised action and running tracks may be a feature. A short muscle-conditioning phase may be included.
Suitable for: Medium to high fitness levels.
Music speed: 145–165 bpm.
Equipment: No equipment required.

High Energy/Impact

Great for those looking to challenge their fitness levels. A large amount of time is devoted to high energy aerobics, and a short segment for developing muscular strength and endurance completes this workout.
Other names: Power Hour, Cardio Hour, Body Blast, Cardio Challenge, Hi Intensity, Aerofit.

Interval Aerobics

Interval classes alternate periods of high intensity cardiovascular work with shorter periods of active recovery. The recovery phase generally incorporates muscle conditioning, non- or low impact exercises and generally lasts for 1.45 mins. The work phase incorporates high and low impact moves and generally lasts for 2.30 mins.
Suitable for: Moderate to high fitness levels.
Music speed: Work 145–165 bpm; active recovery 70–145 bpm.
Equipment: Hand-held weights 2 kg (4–5 lb) or less.

Interval Aerobics

A great class for variety and fun. Interval alternates Hi-Lo segments with a period of active recovery. The recovery is generally a muscle-conditioning phase and allows you to work hard throughout the class due to the varied intensity levels. Suitable for medium to high fitness levels.
Other names: Hi-Lo Interval.

Cross Training

Class consists of three different styles, including Hi-Lo, Low Impact, Interval, Organised Action, Step, Circuits, Body Sculpt, New Body, muscle conditioning and/or flexibility training. Choreography generally lacks complexity and instructors should aim for at least two aerobics-based segments to keep the class flowing.
Suitable for: All fitness levels.
Music speed: Specific to each class format.
Equipment: Hand weights for New Body 2 kg (4–5 lb) or less, or 5 kg (11 lb) or less for Body Sculpt.

Cross Training

Combining three different types of aerobics in the one class. Class components are Hi-Lo, Interval, New Body, Step and/or muscle conditioning. Your instructor will vary the format from week to week and add the element of surprise and fun. A thorough, varied workout.
Other names: Combo Class, CXT, Medley Class, Body Blitz.

Instructor description & guidelines	Consumer description
### Muscle-conditioning Classes Muscle conditioning through the use of such techniques as negative reps, pre-exhaust, blitzing, peripheral heart action, pyramid and reverse pyramid and supersets. Resistance in the form of bands, hand weights, steps and body weight are performed in standing or floor work. Target all muscle groups and maintain intensity levels. **Suitable for:** All fitness levels. **Music speed:** 70–132 bpm. **Equipment:** 5 kg (11 lb) limit for weights, tubes, steps and bands. Resistance should be specific to each individual's level of strength and experience.	### Muscle-conditioning Classes A strong, challenging workout consisting of slow controlled movements with a focus on correct technique and form. Condition your muscles with resistance in the form of body weight, rubberised bands, step platforms and hand weights. A variety of standing and floor exercises will feature in this total body workout. There is no aerobic phase and minimal co-ordination is required. Suitable for any fitness level. **Other names:** Shape Up, Contours, Body Shaping, Body Sculpt.
### New Body Non- or low impact aerobic moves combined with planned upper body conditioning, using light hand held weights. Combinations can be taught with emphasis on simplicity. Encourage form and technique with all armlines. **Suitable for:** All fitness levels. **Music speed:** 70–132 bpm. **Equipment:** Light hand weights 2 kg (4–5 lbs) or lower for less fit participants.	### New Body Non- or low impact aerobics using light hand-held weights. Ideal for upper body conditioning. There is no running or jumping in this class. A great class for both calorie burning and muscle conditioning, with an emphasis on maintaining a lower intensity level for a longer period of time. Suitable for all fitness levels.
### Funk—Stylised Workout Aerobics moves with a definite style, ranging from Street Dance, Funk, City Jam, Latin or Jazz Dance. Great for getting an aerobic workout and for variety. Be aware of the nature of the movements and ensure a thorough warm-up and correct cueing for safety. **Suitable for:** Moderate to high fitness levels. **Music speed:** 127–135 bpm. **Equipment:** No equipment required.	### Funk—Stylised Workout Cardio Funk brings moves from the street, the dance floor and music videos onto the aerobics floor. The music features a great beat to accompany this high-energy workout. A fun class format. **Other names:** Aerofunk, City Jam, Body Jam, Body Beat, Funk, Jazz.

Single- and multi-peak formats

In Low impact, Hi Lo and High Energy classes, two formats have been established.

Single-peak formats

Description: Warm-up, CV phase (travelling, stationary aerobic moves), muscle conditioning, cool-down.

Advantages
- Target heart rates and high energy levels will be achieved in the cardiovascular (CV) phase.
- Intensity can remain consistent in class.
- Fewer format changes throughout class, therefore easier to organise your group.
- Balanced workout consisting of aerobics and muscle isolation in class.
- The body is warmed and well prepared for the muscle-conditioning phase.
- Effective use of overload can be utilised during the muscle-conditioning phase.

Disadvantages
- High stress will be continually placed on the lower body/legs.
- Format of class is predictable and consistent.
- Fatigue may be experienced in the cardiovascular phase. This may result in incorrect form and technique during the CV phase and muscle conditioning.
- It may be difficult for newcomers to maintain high intensity during the CV phase.
- Less variety in class format.

Multi-peak

Description: Warm-up, CV phase, stationary and travelling aerobic moves, muscle conditioning, a CV phase, muscle conditioning, cool-down.

Advantages
- Class format is suitable for beginners to advanced participants.
- Good variety and less continuous stress on the lower body.
- Avoids poor form and technique in muscle conditioning that can be experience after one large CV phase.
- You will not need a large memory bank of exercises or combinations in your planning.

Disadvantages
- If you are not well planned and prepared, the class flow may be lacking.
- Continual transitions to floor or stop/start format may be challenging. This format may require a more experienced instructor.
- Transitions between each phase may be time-consuming.

The most common form of class format is the single-peak class, which will fulfil participants' expectations of getting a 'good CV workout'. The structure of each class is generally dictated by the placement of the muscle-conditioning phase and the length of the cardiovascular phase. Your comfort level, class description and requirements from your centre may dictate the format. Experiment with each format for variety and participant satisfaction level. Request feedback from your participants on class suitability and success of each format.

Class grading systems

The usual forms of class grading systems consist of classification by ability, intensity, and the complexity level of the choreography. The most common of these are the beginner, intermediate and advanced grading of the intensity level. Your participants, both regular and newcomers, should have access to this information on collection of your fitness centre's aerobics timetable. They will be able to place themselves in a suitable class level for comfort, fitness and ability levels, free from frustration and embarrassment. The INTRO performed by the instructor at the start of each class can mention the participants' ability requirements also. All the instructors at your centre should be aware of the grading of each class they teach and the standard the centre sets for the grading. This will make it easier on both participants and instructors.

Grading by intensity level

Beginners	Intermediate	Advanced
Low Intensity	Medium Intensity	High Intensity
Light Pace	Hi-Lo	High Energy

Grading by complexity level

Does the class require you to perform complex choreography or moves, or is it a more athletic basic workout?

Moves — Combinations-based workout. Base moves and their variations will be added together and combined.

Athletic — Less complicated base moves and strong armlines in a freestyle format with little complexity.

Grading by ability or sophistication level

Co-ordination requirement:	A = Low	B = Moderate	C = Challenging
Intensity level:	1 = Low	2 = Medium	3 = High

e.g.
B2	= Medium co-ordination and moderate intensity required.
B1–3	= Moderate co-ordination to suit all levels.
A3	= Low co-ordination and high intensity levels.

Monitoring intensity levels

Three main methods are used when monitoring the intensity levels of your participants. These include:

1. Heart rate checks

A lot of research has been done on heart rate monitoring and training zones. Maximal heart rate can be calculated by using the formula: 220 – age. From this formula, a class participant can establish their training zone, and it is suggested that 70–85% of this maximum figure is accepted as a suitable level for an intermediate class. A newcomer may feel comfortable working within a 60–65% training zone.

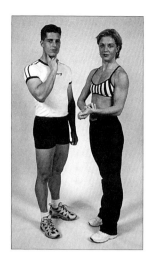

Fig. 12.1. **Heart rate checks**

2. Talk test

A useful tool for immediate observation of participants. Participants should be able to exercise and carry on a conversation at the same time. This indicates that the participant is comfortable with the intensity level. This method requires no special skills or equipment and it can be self-administered.

3. Rating of Perceived Exertion (RPE)

In Table 12.1 a numerical value is applied to a specific rate of exertion. Participants will find their intensity and effort level on the chart to monitor their own intensity level. From this chart they know whether to increase or decrease intensity levels and when to work a little harder or easier. An example of how to use this as a guide may be a rating of 4 as somewhat strong. These charts can usually be found on fitness centre walls for all participants to observe. Educate your participants on the benefits of knowing how hard they are working by using RPE.

0	Nothing at all
1	
2	
3	Moderate
4	
5	Strong
6	
7	Very strong
8	
9	
10	Maximal

Table 12.1. **Rate of Perceived Exertion**

Timetabling

A sample timetable from the Jump and Jive Fitness Centre is given in Table 2.2. The task of timetabling generally lies with the aerobics co-ordinator or manager of the centre. When developing and writing a timetable, the following points need to be considered:

Instructor availability. This should be recorded on a specialised computer program or accessible for all staff. If only one staff member has access to instructor availability, trying to find a replacement instructor can become a lengthy process.

Instructor specialisations or areas of class expertise. Your instructors may feel more confident teaching a certain class style. Ensure that class preferences are also listed with instructor availability.

Variety of instructors. One instructor will find it difficult to front up and teach your participants for the majority of classes week in and week out. Also, your participants need and deserve a variety of styles and instructional techniques. Participants who do follow a particular instructor more than the rest will make time to join their specific classes.

Member feedback. Members may have a preference for a certain instructor. Ensure that you ask a number of participants for their feedback, rather than just the regulars or the front row.

Variety of classes. Try to avoid being known as a Hi-Lo centre or a Circuit centre. Program a variety of classes and instructors each week for the benefits of participant education, awareness and safety aspects of training.

Equipment availability. If your centre owns only 30 step platforms and your 6.30 pm class has a an average regular attendance of 60 participants, there is no point in scheduling a Step class for this time slot. For variety, your centre may create a 50:50 class and timetable two instructors for a Step & Sculpt class at 6.30 pm. Half of the class can work for one interval with the Step instructor and the other half can work with the Sculpt instructor. At the change of each interval, the groups change and the instructors can stay on their respective class formats. Organise your timetable so that classes using the same equipment follow each other, e.g. a Barbell class using steps as benches followed by a Step class. This will reduce the changeover time.

Weekly, bi-weekly or monthly rotating roster— where the class instructor remains the same for a set number of days or weeks. For instructor ease and participant notification, your centre may choose to use either a weekly, bi-weekly or monthly rotating roster. These systems also make it easier for the person who has to write and set the timetable.

Starting and finishing times of classes. What are the busy times within the centre? What class times best cater to your participants' needs and availability? At these busy times, which corresponding instructors and class types does your co-ordinator select to schedule? Will classes be scheduled for 45 minutes or a full hour? These questions and others all need to be considered when planning class times.

Finding replacement instructors. Is it the responsibility of the instructor who is not available to fulfil their teaching duty to find their own replacement, or does that instructor notify the centre within so many hours of their lack of availability? At your centre, whose job is it to find the replacement? Is it up to the person on the counter, the manager, the co-ordinator, or any staff member who is working at the time? What if an instructor is expected to teach a class and, without any notice, they do not show up? What emergency procedures are in place?

Timetable advertising, distribution of timetables and centre displays. Printed timetables for the month can be distributed to members either with or without the instructors' names listed. It may be easier to train your members to come for classes rather than for an instructor.

Aerobics class budget within the centre. How many classes can each full-time instructor teach vs part-time or freelance instructors? What does each class cost

JUMP AND JIVE FITNESS CENTRE TIMETABLE						
Times	Mon	Tues	Wed	Thur	Fri	Sat
6.30 am	Circuit		Step Athletic		Hi-Lo	
9.30 am	Step Athletic	New Body	Hi-Lo	Sculpt	Body Pump	X-Train
1.00 pm	Hi-Lo	Step Athletic	Circuit	Step Athletic	Sculpt	
4.30 pm	Step	Body Pump	Kids Club	Box Circuit	New Body	
5.30 pm	Hi-Lo	X-Train	Step Athletic	Body Pump	Hi-Lo	
6.30 pm	Step Moves	Interval	Body Pump	Low Impact	Stretch	
7.30 pm	New Body	Step Intro	Lite Pace	X-Train		

YOUR FITNESS CENTRE TIMETABLE						
Times	Mon	Tues	Wed	Thur	Fri	Sat

Table 12.2. **Timetables**

the centre? How many casual members does the centre need to attend each class to break even? How much money each week does your centre allocate for aerobics classes? These factors must be discussed with the centre manager or owner and clearly stated before the timetable is set. More information on the role of the aerobics co-ordinator is given in Chapter 14.

Considerations

- Jump and Jive is a busy suburban fitness centre. The emphasis has always been on member education and the awareness of staying motivated through variety, challenge and fun. The members range from teenagers to retired pensioners, with the majority of members ranging from 25–45 years.
- Clientele include 6.30 am regulars who like variety and change. They are more frequent on Monday, Wednesday and Friday. There is a large membership base of mothers who take advantage of free child-minding from 9–11 am Monday to Saturday.
- A corporate base frequents the lunchtime classes. They come and go at different times during this hour but enjoy variety to ensure that they get a total body workout each week.
- Kids' fitness is a big part of the Wednesday timetable, with free child-minding being offered from 5.30–8.00 pm on Wednesday evenings.
- An older group of newcomers who attend later in the evenings, after mealtimes, are interested in being led in class by an instructor. 7.30 pm classes are the least attended, with 5.30 pm and 6.30 pm the most popular. The 4.30 pm class is well attended by teenagers, students and shift workers.
- The Step and Body Pump by Les Mills© programs are frequented by members. There are regular requests for additional classes.
- Equipment. The centre is well equipped with steps, barbells, hand weights, resistance bands and slides.
- Equipment and efficiency of class changeover. Body Pump by Les Mills© is followed by Step, or vice versa, to reduce equipment set-up time.

✗ ✗ Drill ✗ ✗

Use Jump and Jive Fitness Centre as a model and design a timetable for your centre.

Special Populations

The pregnant exerciser

Regular exercise and muscle conditioning during pregnancy will give the 'mum-to-be' more energy during her pregnancy and more strength to look after her baby afterwards. When done properly and with supervision to accommodate the ever-changing body, exercise programs can counteract some of the shoulder and back pain than can be caused by growing breasts and an enlarging uterus. Every pregnant body and every pregnancy will be different; it is therefore inappropriate for an instructor to take the responsibility of prescribing prenatal exercise programs without a physician's approval.

First to third trimester

Obvious trimester changes and considerations are: increased body mass, joint laxity, postural realignment, generalised fatigue and increased cardiovascular demands. Resting oxygen consumption increases gradually to approximately 20–30% above prepregnancy level in the third trimester. Resting HR increases approximately 7 bpm in first trimester, peaking at approx. 15 bpm above the prepregnancy rate near third trimester. Average pregnancy weight gains are between about 12 and 15 kgs (27 to 34 lbs); body fat increases an average of 4 to 5%. (ACOG, 1994.)

The following is a summary of the American College of Obstetricians and Gynaecologists (ACOG) guidelines for exercise in pregnancy and post-partum. As long as you don't have any additional risk factors, ACOG suggests that you:

- Continue an exercise regimen during pregnancy. A regular program, at least three times a week, is preferable to random workouts.
- Stop exercising in the supine position after the first trimester. It can decrease your heart's output to the uterus. Also, avoid standing motionless for a prolonged period.

- Stop exercising when you're fatigued, and never push to exhaustion. If you don't have problems, you may be able to continue weight-bearing exercises at the same intensity as you did before pregnancy, but non–weight-bearing exercises, such as cycling or swimming, may be easier to do and present less risk of injury.
- Avoid exercise that has the potential for even mild abdominal trauma. Also, be careful of exercises in which your growing belly might affect your balance (and lead to falls), especially in the third trimester.
- Make sure your diet is adequate. Pregnant women require 300 additional calories a day if they are exercising.
- Be careful to stay cool while exercising in the first trimester: Drink a lot of water, wear appropriate clothing and avoid overheated environments. Take your temperature if necessary, as the foetus is fragile during the early stages of development. Ensure a toilet is nearby, as frequent urination can be common.
- Resume your pre-pregnancy exercise routines gradually after giving birth. Pregnancy's physical changes persist for four to six weeks post-partum.

The conditions that preclude exercise during pregnancy, as advised by ACOG, are shown in Table 13.1.

Absolute contraindications	Relative contraindications
Pregnancy-induced hypertension	Breech presentation in the last trimester
Pre-term membrane ruptures	History of extremely sedentary lifestyle
Previous or current pre-term labour	Extremely underweight
A surgically closed or incompetent cervix	Persistent second or third trimester bleeding
Retarded intrauterine growth	Hypertension
History of three or more spontaneous miscarriages	Anaemia
Diagnosed multiple pregnancies	Thyroid disease
Placenta praevia (placenta is implanted in the lower uterine segment, making it vulnerable to detachment)	Diabetes

Table 13.1. **Absolute and relative contraindications to exercise during pregnancy***

Designing a prenatal exercise class

When designing prenatal classes, the best guidelines that we can follow are those from the American College of Obstetricians and Gynaecologists (ACOG) and the American College of Sports Medicine (ACSM). In 1994 ACOG released an updated, research-based technical bulletin, 'Exercise During Pregnancy and the Postpartum Period'. Gone now are the heart rate and exercise duration limitations, and in their place there are realistic and adaptive guidelines for each pregnant woman. Human data 'indicates a pregnant woman can exercise safely with minimal risk to herself and her fetus', according to ACSM researchers.

- A doctor's certificate from your client or participant should be your first requirement. Make sure the mother-to-be has carefully discussed her exercise program with her doctor.
- Exercise should be stopped immediately if your pregnant participant feels very hot, faint, dizzy, has shortness of breath, experiences vaginal bleeding, palpitations, blurred vision, disorientation, or has a continuous or severe headache. Exercise should be also be stopped if there are feelings of lower abdominal pain, back or pubic pain.
- A long warm-up period of 10–15 minutes should be performed. This allows for a gradual progression into the cardiovascular phase.
- The cardiovascular phase should be for a maximum of 15–20 minutes and can be taught in a multi-peak format (see Chapter 12) to allow for recovery periods to rest and cool the body.
- A long recovery period (5–10 mins) should follow the cardiovascular phase.
- No exercises, or a very limited number of exercises, should be performed in the prone or supine positions.
- Exercise should be performed on a wooden floor or a tightly carpeted floor to reduce impact forces.
- Hand weights should be no heavier than 0.5 kg (1 lb) as this can rapidly elevate the heart rate. No rubberised resistance should be used around the lower limbs, as this may restrict blood flow.
- Extreme flexion or extension of joints and activities that require jumps, jarring or rapid changes in

direction should be avoided. This is because the hormone relaxin, which is released during pregnancy, causes connective tissue laxity and may result in joint instability.
- In order to strengthen the pelvic floor, Kegel exercises that involve contracting the muscles used to shut off the flow of urine, should be performed. Each contraction should last for 5–10 seconds and they can be performed when stretching or doing muscle conditioning exercises throughout the class.
- Emphasise stretching and the associated relaxation. Avoid any ballistic (bouncy or jerky) movements.

Evaluating and testing intensity levels

Pregnant women may have lower workout capacities, and the conventional methods of determining exercise intensity HR testing may be inappropriate because of an increase in the expectant mother's resting heart rate between first and third trimesters. Because of this, a combination of rate of perceived exertion (RPE) and pulse rates is better for determining intensity levels.

Incorporating pregnant exercisers into a conventional class

When a specialty pregnancy class is not available in your centre, there are many ways for you to incorporate a mother-to-be into your regular classes. The guidelines above can also be used when instructing your classes.

- Ensure that she has a permission letter from her doctor to exercise.
- Encourage her to stand to the front but to the side of the class, so that you can monitor her intensity and she can adequately view you to follow the class.
- If your pregnant participant hasn't exercised before, start very slowly or wait one trimester. If she has been a frequent exerciser, don't increase the level of exercise.
- Encourage her to take continual drink breaks and monitor her body temperature. Comfortable loose clothing should be worn, with a supportive bra to cater for enlarging and possibly tender breasts.

Variations of exercises in the prone and supine positions should be demonstrated as an alternative. If the music or movements become faster, or direction changes become more rapid, your pregnant exerciser should know that she can modify any of the movements being performed. An alternative to hi-impact moves should also be demonstrated. Gentle stretching should be encouraged in the cool-down.

Seniors

Slowly becoming one of the largest population groups, over-50s or seniors are estimated to represent 20% of the total population by the year 2000. This group is having a large influence on the fitness industry and, to cater for their needs, fitness centres are developing a wide range of specific programs and services.

When classifying or grading senior exercise classes, mobility and activity levels are always considered before age. Although grading by age groups simply refers to over 50s, or over 60s, this can be an inappropriate grading system as some 50-year-olds are far more active than their 30-year-old counterparts. We have chosen to grade them as semi-mobile and active mobile.

1. **Semi-mobile:** These participants are not chair-bound but do require some form of walking assistance.
2. **Active mobile:** Participants in this grade generally have full range of motion in all limbs, and can walk unaided.

General guidelines for semi-mobile and active mobile seniors

- Easy and gradual warm-up, with emphasis on full ROM.
- Avoid all ballistic, bouncy or jarring movements on upper and lower limbs.
- Limit 'above the head' armlines, as these can increase blood pressure.
- When using hand weights, keep the limit 0.5 kg (1 lb).
- Because of the variation in heart rates due to age, medication and activity levels, RPE will be the most appropriate gauge of intensity and comfort level.
- Encourage comfortable, layered clothing that can easily be removed in humid weather.

- Participants should drink plenty of fluids before, during and after their workout.
- Participants should be able to easily complete the class and have a great sense of achievement when finished. Try to finish on a high, with a positive comment, statement, activity or drill.

Semi-mobile

These participants are more concerned with health-related gains than with physical appearance or looks. Members of this group tend to use sticks, frames or wheelchairs to aid their mobility and they are generally older than the active mobile. Many may be on medication for arthritis, hypertension, diabetes, heart disorders or other age-related conditions.

The class

Due to their mobility level, the class may be conducted at the group's place of residence (e.g. nursing home, day care centre) or the group may have a set class and arrive together by bus to your fitness centre.

The focus of the class will be on mobility, circulation improvement, muscle tone, co-ordination, interaction, fun and self-esteem.

The use of a bar will be helpful to this group to support standing exercises; alternatively, many standing exercises can be adapted so that they can be performed in a seated position. This group generally doesn't like to get down and exercise on the floor.

Exercises are limited for this group and they may fatigue faster than the active mobile group. Therefore, it is suggested that class times range from 25–40 minutes.

Warm-up: Easy seated ROM exercises 3–5 mins with a light stretch 2–3 mins.

Conditioning: Slowly build up to more medium to advanced isolated and combination seated exercises or standing routines that last for 15–20 mins. Encourage interaction and ensure that the music selected is not too loud and is appropriate to the age group.

Cool-down: Slowly reduce the intensity levels by using easy ROM exercises and a possible chair stretch of 3–5 mins. A common song or fun armline routine can be incorporated into this session.

Relaxation techniques: 2–3 mins.

Active mobile

This group has more time and money to spend on themselves and their health. They are concerned with their self-image, appearance and self esteem. They would be capable of joining into a low impact style class, but may be turned off by the loud music or they may perceive it to be too strenuous. They may also object to participating in a class named 'Over 50s', as they still feel they are active and youthful and do not like being 'branded'. These classes can be named appropriately to suit the group or even named by the group itself, e.g. 'The swingers class' or 'Energise hour'.

The class

A single peak format should be followed, similar to low-impact aerobics, for approximately 45 minutes in total. Fun partner activities and dances can be incorporated into this class format and flexibility work should be included.

Warm-up: 5 mins
Conditioning: 30–35 mins
Cool-down: 5–10 mins

A decision to include muscle conditioning on the floor would take into consideration the following points: the benefits of variety, strength and muscle conditioning vs mobility considerations, hypertension and modesty. Evaluate and screen your group to aid in assessing the best class options.

The instructor's role

- **Attitude.** A positive, empathetic attitude is essential. Encourage your participants, create an instructor image that they can respect. Have fun: you must enjoy the class and really show it!
- **Form.** Full ROM should be encouraged without over-extension. Make it comfortable for participants to work at their own pace. Your form should be correct yet relaxed throughout the class.
- **Cueing.** As some participants may have loss of visual and hearing abilities, a combination of verbal and visual cues will be required. These cues should be clear, simple and to the point. Watch your use of 'slang' or modern terms when cueing or encouraging your participants. Allow them to feel relaxed, and confident that they can easily follow and understand you.

- **Know your participants.** Ensure that all participants follow a pre-screening assessment and have medical clearances before participating in classes. Learn what complaints or conditions your participants have, and know what to expect from signs and symptoms. Keep a watchful eye on your group at all times.
- **Music.** Music has always been significant to any generation. Choose appropriate songs that reflect the era of your participants. Some examples may include square-dancing tunes, polkas, Latin rhythms, cha chas, early Beach Boys, Frank Sinatra songs, big band classics, etc.

A very special person—one with qualities far greater than those of a regular instructor—will have a great deal of fun teaching this group. Ensure a good technical base is established, and a sensible approach to the importance of this class. You will have a positive impact on the quality of life that your classes can bring to this group.

Children

There is a definite need for formal children's exercise classes. Cardiovascular fitness, strength and flexibility are an important part of children's exercise classes and their general development. In addition to this, gross motor skills, co-ordination, self-expression, imagination, balance, rhythm and teamwork are all important class considerations. This class is much more than a mini-adult workout. It needs to be a unique and special occasion for all children.

Children can be classified into two main groups: Early childhood from 3–7 years, and Pre-adolescent from 7–12 years. Programs should emphasise the goal of non-competitive fitness and skill development, with an emphasis on participation and fun.

'But children are so active—why do they need formal exercise programs?' you ask. Consider the following statistics:
- Schools are reducing physical education and daily exercise curricula.
- Fitness is at its lowest level for children. Recent studies have discovered that children whose counterparts 10 years ago could do 10 press ups, could only manage 4 in the same time today.
- Childhood obesity is at the highest level (one in three 12–16-year-olds are obese, and one in two 12–16-year-olds have high cholesterol).
- Self-esteem is the lowest and teenage suicide rates are at their highest levels.
- Participation in competitive sport is declining.
- Many children possess one or even more coronary heart-disease risk factors.

With this in mind, look at the following acronym for KIDS:

Keep them moving.
Imagination—always allow children to express themselves.
Diversity—ensure optimal variety in programming, for shorter attention span and motivation levels.
Self esteem—always be positive with children. Build their confidence in their own abilities, their skills and their interaction with other children.

Early childhood and pre-adolescent considerations

- Make it fun and have fun yourself. Children always know when you are faking it!
- Classes will run for approximately 30 minutes, depending on attention spans, with a gradual increase and decrease in intensity levels for both warm-ups and cool-downs.
- Avoid the overuse of any one activity and continual high-impact moves.
- Plan thoroughly, including alternatives. Always be prepared for change if your activities aren't working.
- Encourage drink breaks throughout the workout, and light clothing in humid weather.
- Never use exercise as a punishment; reinforce all the positive aspects of exercise.

3–7-year-olds

Focus on fun and enjoyment, with fitness being a hidden benefit. This group is experiencing rapid growth and mind development. Fun but challenging games should be included in classes that focus on imagery. Minimal complexity with choreography or routines should be attempted. All routines should be fun and enjoyable.

7–12-year-olds

Fewer games should be used with this group. Always aim the imagery components much higher, due to the influence of music trends and fashion on this group. Choreography can be included in the class, with an emphasis on co-ordination or cross co-ordination development (where necessary).

Include some educational tips to create awareness of health, fitness, nutrition and incorporating exercise into their weekly routines. Fun and enjoyment is still a focus of classes. As the children are getting older, fitness becomes an emphasised benefit. To increase their fitness level, more intensity can be encouraged with each activity. This is a critical age, where children will develop their own ideas on exercise. Always aim to create a positive and enjoyable environment!

Marketing tips for special populations

The ability of a fitness club and its instructors to cater for special populations will be a benefit to any organisation. These classes can be advertised to the existing membership base, their families and friends, the local community, nursing homes, community groups or organisations such as senior citizens, prenatal clinics at the local hospitals and local schools.

Children's activities cannot exist without parents or carers bringing the children to the centre—these adults may be interested in joining in some activity at the same time. When establishing programs for special populations, a fitness centre must have well-trained and qualified staff who have the right personality and enthusiasm to handle each group. This will ensure the continued success and longevity of these classes and programs.

Professional Development

As an instructor, you are expected to possess many qualities and attributes. You will be a role model, adviser and friend to your group. Unfortunately, some instructors believe success is based on how fit they look and on their technical skills. This is very different to an employer's and, indeed, a participant's perspective.

The qualities of a great instructor

The great instructor is no ordinary person. In or out of the fitness profession, this individual possesses the qualities that mark a special human being. The great instructor is empathetic, happy, energetic, enthusiastic, motivated, skilful, compassionate, sincere, encouraging, honest, approachable, reliable, neat and tidy, confident, dedicated, professional, organised, accommodating and consistent. In addition, this person is a born leader, with a healthy physical appearance and possessing individuality, versatility, musicality and a good sense of humour. And, because he/she is an effective communicator, the great instructor is an inspiring teacher.

More specifically, the great aerobics instructor:

- Genuinely wants to improve the health and fitness of participants; shows empathy and sincere care for participants.
- Genuinely wants to contribute to the business success of their employer.
- Can communicate on and off the aerobics floor and stage area.
- Is punctual and is well prepared before the class.
- Is a good resource and advisory person for participants and peers.
- Is a skilled observer.
- Leads by example and sells the benefits of health and fitness.
- Always presents with a neat and professional attire.
- Is aware of participants' needs/wants and is able to plan classes accordingly.
- Always varies their music selection.

- Maintains a high standard of education and knowledge.
- Knows their own threshold for giving 100% effort, energy and consistency.
- Is realistic and aware of their own skill and ability level.

Now that we have met the ideal instructor, let us examine other important aspects of his/her professional life.

Evaluations

Evaluations are an important part of instructing. You have an obligation to your participants, your centre and to yourself to ensure that your performance is the best it can be. Constructive criticism will help you to improve, maintain quality and consistent standards when teaching.

Evaluations can occur on three levels: i) participant evaluation, ii) self evaluation and iii) peer evaluation, for example by the aerobics co-ordinator. The most common of these will be self-evaluation.

Self-awareness is a vital personal skill. Evaluate your good and bad points effectively. For example, do you always watch your participants on one side rather than equally on both? Are you overusing the same words in your classes? Is your terminology and exercise vocabulary correct? Are you presenting a professional image? Are you really making an effort to meet your participants and learn their names? Are you as motivated as you should be during your classes? Is it time for you to have a short break to recover in order to be a great teacher? Is it time for an update? Effective self-evalution will help to make you a great instructor.

Evaluations provide meaningful feedback and valuable information, but they can be stressful. To take the stress and nervousness out of instructor evaluations, try these simple tips:

- **Regularity.** Ask your fellow staff, co-ordinator and participants to evaluate you regularly. Ensure that these are people whose opinion you respect and trust.
- **Share and grow.** Evaluations allow you to share ideas and grow professionally. They are not used to create competition or direct criticism.
- **Plus and minus.** Focus on positive aspects of performance and improve your weaknesses. Support all of your fellow staff and management in their decision to evaluate and improve.
- **New methods.** When asking your group for feedback on music used, have participants vote with their feet, or by moving to different ends of the room according to satisfaction or dissatisfaction levels.
- **Formal feedback.** Have your participants, instructors and management complete a formalised written feedback or evaluation form.
- **Self-awareness.** Evaluate yourself after each and every class. You can be your own best and severest critic. Learn to identify your own strengths and weaknesses; quietly celebrate your improvements, and recognise where you need to improve.
- **Be appreciative.** Feedback and evaluations can be difficult for all concerned. You should be grateful to any participant or fellow staff for their assistance. Ensure that you thank all involved, whether the comments are positive or negative.

Goal setting

Have an action plan. After an evaluation, set yourself goals to improve, and then be re-evaluated.

Always be realistic with your goal setting. Set both short- and long-term professional and personal goals for yourself. An example of a realistic short-term goal may be to work for two weeks on mastering music phrasing. Practise as often as possible. Listen to as many pieces of music as possible. Work on your drills with a partner and by yourself. Practise your music maps, etc. After this goal has been achieved, work for two weeks on developing another teaching skill.

Drill

Continually evaluate yourself—you will be your own most critical judge. Draw up a schedule with two columns headed 'Strengths' and 'Weaknesses', and list all your positives and negatives—but avoid too much emphasis on the negatives. Ask a close friend or instructor whom you respect to evaluate you once a month, or request an instructor evaluation by the fitness centre management.

Participant expectations

Continually seek feedback and comments from your participants on their likes and dislikes. Participants can certainly make our job a difficult one at times but, realistically, all participants are at your centre for one or more of the following reasons:

- to improve their overall health and fitness;
- to lose body fat/weight management;
- for medical/health reasons;
- to improve muscle strength and endurance;
- to socialise;
- to reduce stress;
- injury recovery/prevention;
- to have fun.

To learn more about what makes your clientele tick, approach your centre manager about conducting a formal survey to ascertain participants' likes and dislikes.

Staying motivated

'Instructor burnout' can occur through inadequate diet, physical fatigue, not keeping up-to-date, no holidays for an extended time period, or many years in the industry.

Here are some sure signs that you may need to reassess your teaching schedule and work on strategies to modify what you are doing. Identifying these factors may be all it takes to remotivate and reactivate yourself.

- Irritability with participants.
- Sudden drop in performance.
- Difficulty in sleeping.
- Irritability, short temper and depression.
- Increase in resting heart rate.
- Muscle fatigue and cramping.
- Permanent feeling of tiredness.
- Lack of motivation.
- Loss of appetite, anaemia or oedema.
- Amenorrhoea.
- Overuse soft-tissue injuries, tendonitis, shin splints.
- Voice complaints or vocal injuries.

To overcome or avoid 'instructor burnout' you may need to cut back on the number of classes you are teaching each week, take a break altogether, change the class style you are teaching regularly, purchase new music, attend an aerobics workshop or convention, watch a training video, find another hobby outside of the fitness industry, or attend another instructor's class for a change. These simple tips may be all you need to get you back on track fast!

One sure tactic for recharging your batteries is to attend a workshop or convention.

Continuing education

In many countries, instructors have to show proof of continuing education to maintain their certification. When attending a single- or multi-day event, ensure that you are well prepared to take advantage of it. Set yourself goals, take business cards to network with fellow professionals, ask questions, take notes, and write your own descriptions or interpretation of moves or lectures so that you can fully understand this information after the event is over. Attend a variety of sessions so that your overall knowledge can be improved.

Don't always attend events just for an aerobics update. Try attending a nutrition seminar or communication workshop to enhance your overall knowledge and skills, and to keep abreast of the industry. Have a positive attitude and make the most of every opportunity!

The role of the aerobics co-ordinator

After you have had several years of experience as an instructor, you may be interested in pursuing a co-ordinating or managerial role within your centre or another centre. Listed below are the duties and responsibilities in which an aerobics co-ordinator will need to be competent in order to perform a successful role within a centre. Do you fit the job?

The aerobics co-ordinator's most important tasks are:

1. Tracking class numbers and meeting minimums.
2. Tracking participant satisfaction and meeting minimum levels.

Others include:
- Recruiting, hiring instructors.
- Training new instructors on club policies, rules and standards.
- Training existing instructors to ensure that all staff remain updated, qualified and professional through in-house workshops and 'jam' sessions.
- Preparing the aerobics timetable—instructor availability, class times, class types, current trends and member satisfaction (see Chapter 12 for further timetabling information).
- Conducting instructor evaluations and feedback.
- Purchasing of musical tapes, or advising staff in this area.
- Developing and continually enforcing the health and safety policies of the fitness club.
- Educating members through seminars, handouts and newsletters.
- Organising member motivational classes and programs, such as theme classes or evenings.
- Teaching a certain number of classes within the centre each week, and participating in other instructors' classes.
- Keeping yourself updated by attending workshops, conventions and seminars.
- Maintaining your own fitness level and health.
- Liaising between instructors and management with direct feedback, by attending meetings or preparing reports.
- Preparing a demonstration team and routine for external or internal promotions.
- Giving participants the opportunity to provide feedback on classes, instructors and centre operations.
- Providing feedback to instructors from management and participants.

Employment issues

Seeking employment in this diverse and challenging industry requires that you be well prepared. This segment of the chapter outlines some of the necessary steps you will need to consider. Aerobics instructing is a profession, so treat your job with respect and dignity.

Getting the job

Replying to an advertisement

Always type your reply (and print it on good quality paper), develop a powerful résumé, and know the name of the person who will be conducting the interview. All correspondence should be directed to that person. In addition to a standard résumé, you can include a head-shot photo.

Your résumé

This should include your personal details, all past and current employment, education history, presentations, awards, achievements, professional affiliations and the names of at least three referees who are familiar with your experience in the industry. Your résumé should be no more than two typed pages covering the major aspects of your professional career.

An opening or cover letter should be included to express interest in the position advertised, and to request an interview. If your background of awards and affiliations requires more space than your two-page résumé allows, you may wish to state in your cover letter that you will be glad to provide these details at an interview.

Copies of relevant certificates should be included to support your application. If you gain an interview take the originals with you, but never allow these valuable professional documents to leave your possession.

Do your homework

Research the centre, as this will present you as a professional with a sincere interest in the job. Your knowledge of the centre and its style will impress the interviewer and give you a head start over other applicants. Join into an aerobics class at the centre, if possible, to see if the club specialises in any class style or if the formats differ from your regular classes. This will also allow you to assess the current instructor's ability levels. Talk to some centre members and find out if there are any current problems at the centre that they may need new staff to help solve; you may also hear about new programs, or an expansion period in the near future.

The interview

When selected for a job interview, remember that the interview does not commence when you enter the door of the centre, but way before then. Plan for your interview, know what to expect, learn all you can about the centre, the position, the clientele, and always follow up the day after the interview.

Here are some sample questions. Write your response to each question to prepare yourself for the interview.

Preparation

Q1 What skills have you developed that you can offer to our club?
Q2 What are your strengths?
Q3 What are your weaknesses?
Q4 Why are you changing jobs? *or* Why did you leave your last job?
Q5 What interests you about this position?
Q6 Under what conditions do you work best?
Q7 Do you enjoy working by yourself or with others?
Q8 What are your areas of interest or class specialisation?
Q9 What other concepts could you bring to our centre?
Q10 What are your long-term career goals as an instructor?

Always expand on each question. Don't be afraid to ask the interviewer to repeat a question or explain it if you are unsure of what they expect from your answer. Always demonstrate your motivation and enthusiasm for the position.

After the interview

Take time to write a thank-you or follow-up letter to your interviewer. If you were unsuccessful in obtaining the position, call once a month to let the centre know that you are still available if any other positions arise. Join into classes at the centre to make yourself known to participants and staff.

What to wear

Prepare for the interview in two ways. Look professional for a seated interview, prepare for an audition. Convey that you are serious about the job from the start by creating a positive first impression. For an audition you will normally be asked to teach a full class, teach components of a class, attend a centre training session or join a class taught by your interviewer. Practice for this audition. Go through your INTRO, even if you are just demonstrating to the interviewer. Have your music ready and take time to familiarise yourself with the sound system. Your selected outfit should be clean, relatively new and fitted. Shoes and socks should be clean and tidy. Your hair should be neat and both men and women should ensure that they have adequate support by selecting an appropriate bra for women or a dance support for men.

The Facility

This chapter outlines the necessities and requirements of an aerobics facility. If you are interested in establishing, designing or creating your own aerobics business, or are commissioned to do so by a fitness club, the guidelines listed below will be useful.

Always contact your local government authority to check with standards and guidelines.

It's always a good idea to check other facilities for ideas and feedback. Ask as many questions as you can to make sure you are happy with your choices.

The aerobics room — Standards and guidelines

Following are the important questions to answer when designing or evaluating your facility:

- Is it a single- or multi-purpose room? Will the room be used for aerobics-based programs only, or will it be used for other activities, e.g. dance classes, circuit classes, seminars, social events?
- Is the environment safe and free from unreasonable hazards?
- Is it well ventilated?
- Is it aesthetically appealing?
- Is it clean?
- Are drinking water and rest rooms close by?
- How many participants will you comfortably fit into this area?
- Will your area have a freestanding ceiling or will there be pillars or columns throughout the floor space?
- Is there a clear emergency exit in and out of this area large enough to accommodate your group of participants?

These and other questions are all factors to consider.

The following facility standards and guidelines serve as an easily followed guide for the facility and for participant safety. Additional guidelines are outlined in the American College of Sports Medicine's *Health/Fitness Facility Standards and Guidelines*.

- Equipment should be well maintained, regularly checked, cleaned and, above all, safe.
- Air-handling systems must be established that control air pressure and air into the facility.
- Each participant should have at least 4–4.5 metres (11–12 feet) of space for each session, and the minimum ceiling height needs to be 3 metres (8 feet).
- Mirrors need to be provided on at least two of the four walls, starting from 15 cm (6 in) off the floor to the ceiling.
- Impact absorption floors should be installed in either wood or carpet. The underlay should be sufficient to absorb impact created by the users.
- Walls can be insulated to avoid sound travelling outside of this area.
- An adequate sound system should be provided in the aerobics area.
- Additional equipment should be provided to enhance participation within the aerobics room. This includes exercise mats, tubes, bands and hand held weights, benches and/or steps.
- Temperature should range from 19–22 degrees Celsius (68–72 degrees Fahrenheit).
- Humidity should be 60% or less.
- Air circulation: 8–12 exchanges per hour.
- There should be adequate natural and/or artificial lighting throughout the room.
- Sound levels: 70–80 decibels.

Floor-space requirements

For safety and practicality, your participants need a large enough training area to have suitable personal space in which to exercise comfortably. This will ensure that any type of injuries from contact or collision will be minimised. As mentioned before, each participant should have at least 4–4.5 metres (11–12 feet) of space for each session, and the minimum ceiling height needs to be 3 metres (8 feet).

Floor designs will differ in relation to the space available to you, whether you are in rented, previously built accommodation or a purpose-built facility.

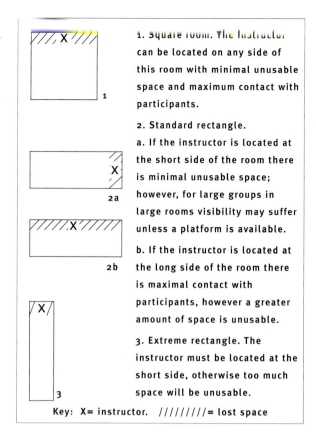

1. Square room. The instructor can be located on any side of this room with minimal unusable space and maximum contact with participants.

2. Standard rectangle.
   a. If the instructor is located at the short side of the room there is minimal unusable space; however, for large groups in large rooms visibility may suffer unless a platform is available.
   b. If the instructor is located at the long side of the room there is maximal contact with participants, however a greater amount of space is unusable.

3. Extreme rectangle. The instructor must be located at the short side, otherwise too much space will be unusable.

Key: X= instructor. ///////= lost space

Fig. 15.1. **Common floor designs**

An important decision when designing your aerobics floor is whether to have an open vs a closed room. Will the room be open for all other activities and exercisers to view the aerobics participants? Will the room be enclosed or secluded from the view of other exercisers?

This decision is one that may affect the type of clientele your facility will attract. Deconditioned clients may feel threatened and intimidated by exercising in front of 'interested onlookers'. Females may wish to exercise away from male view. For a young and fit clientele, these points may not even be a consideration or concern.

Floor type and maintenance

The choice of flooring is a major consideration when selecting or designing an aerobics room. Check all requirements before investing in your flooring.

The two most common floor types for the aerobics room are: (i) sprung wooden flooring and (ii) carpet on underlay.

Sprung wooden flooring has been designed to reduce impact and shock to the joints by minimising the effects of impact. However, wooden floors may be slippery when wet with perspiration or water. This floor needs to be washed regularly. If a cleaning product is required, this should be tested to ensure it does not make the floor slippery; vacuuming between washes will assist with general cleanliness and care of this flooring. Mats will be required for participants.

If laid on concrete, carpet requires a high-quality underlay. The specialty underlay greatly reduces the impact forces and the carpet is generally softer when participants are doing any type of floor work. Carpet has a firm traction for participants when making quick direction changes. Obviously, carpet will wear more quickly than wooden flooring, and it will require regular cleaning. Sweat will be absorbed into the carpet and slowly change its appearance and quality. It is more difficult to see hair and dust on carpet, as opposed to wooden flooring; however, regular vacuuming of either surface will assist with general maintenance.

When cleaning carpets in your facility, select a dry-cleaning option over steam cleaning. Steam cleaning takes a lot longer to dry, and it can shrink certain carpet brands.

Once again, check all requirements before investing in your flooring.

Instructing platform

Small rooms may not require a platform, but medium and large rooms will need an instructor platform. When building a platform, consider the amount of space that certain aerobic moves use when travelling. The execution of such moves as 8 marches fwd or bwd, a double grapevine, etc. takes a lot of space.

Take care when deciding on the height of the platform. It should be possible for the instructor to move freely from it to interact with participants, but at the same time it must be high enough for clients in the back row to see the instructor's foot patterns.

Sound systems

For starters you will need an amplifier, a single or twin tape deck with pitch control and a microphone output system. A back-up or replacement sound system is a must for any facility.

The speakers should be of reasonable quality—know their capabilities and soundwave patterns. The speakers should be placed off the floor to carry the best sound throughout your room. Avoid cheap, home stereo speakers as these will not deliver the quality sound your participants expect.

To get the right location for your speakers and sound system, have an expert sound technician assist with your decision making. There is a definite need for positive acoustics in your room. (For more information on sound equipment see Chapter 2.)

The class— Standards and guidelines

- Participants should be adequately screened before participating in exercise classes.
- Attendance should be recorded for aerobics sessions and a variety of class styles should be offered at each centre to cater for different needs and wants.
- A written schedule of the timetable should be provided so that participants can better plan their exercise efforts each week.
- Instructors should have required qualifications to ensure participant safety.
- There must be ready access to water facilities to replace fluids, and to men's and women's locker rooms and toilets.
- Participants should not enter during a class unless they have warmed up.
- Participants should always wear appropriate clothing and footwear.

Random checks should be conducted in the centre on your instructors, the equipment and participants to ascertain that these standards and guidelines are being adhered to.

Signage

Advertising your aerobics program should be a high priority for management and for each instructor. Signs inside the club are one of the most effective promotional tools. All signs, especially the timetable, should be placed in public access for maximum exposure.

As your timetable may change every week or month, it is important to ensure that your signage meets a professional standard. It needs to be determined what information each sign is meant to provide, and the intended audience. Consideration should be made regarding the attractiveness of each sign. The colours should match the facility and should catch the reader's eye. If aerobic signs are handwritten, they should be neat and in the one handwriting. Don't allow each of your instructors to make corrections to the signs, keep the writing consistent. The writing should be large enough to read from 2 metres (6–7 feet) away.

Any symbols on the aerobic signs need to be identified and defined, e.g. grading for classes may be shown by asterisks as follows: * beginners; ** intermediate; *** advanced. If these asterisks are displayed on the timetable, they must be included with class descriptions and ability levels. General signs within the aerobics area need to highlight the location of drinking water within the facility and male/female changing-room signs need to be visible.

All signs need to be placed at a readable height for your participants. Eye level is a general guide for placement and optimal visibility, however placement height for disabled members will differ from this. Do not place signs close to each other. Prioritise signs and their placement within your centre.

Storage of equipment

When storing aerobics equipment, consider the safety of your participants and conservation of space. All equipment storage within the aerobics area needs to be tidy and out of harm's way. Your aerobics room needs to be set up so that participants can make full use of the space. You will not be able to accommodate many participants in a tightly packed aerobics room. Storage of equipment and ease of accessibility will always be a special consideration.

Barbells can be stored upright along the walls in a set stand. Special barbell racks can be obtained to store both bars and weights.

Steps should be stacked neatly against a wall. The traditional step platforms should be stacked end-to-end and top-to-bottom, and the new platforms should be stacked no more than six steps high. This allows for easy access and allows for participant height variations.

Hand weights should be stored in a container or on a rack for ease of selection. If stored in a container, ensure that there are at least two containers apart from each other for easy access. Plan your group organisation carefully if your hand weights are stored in one location. Hand weights should be cleaned regularly to ensure that the grips are not too worn or affected by participants' sweat. This may cause the hand weight to rust over a period of time. If your hand weights are painted, have your instructors request that participants should not bang or tap the weights together, as this will remove the paint and make the floor dirty.

Rubberised resistance should be stored in a container that allows air circulation to assist in drying. If participants tie a strip band into a circle, it should be untied before storage. Bands with handles may be hung in an area of the aerobics room, or a storage bag can be used for all rubberised resistance. Check when purchasing your bands for maintenance tips such as cleaning or powdering. Regularly check the bands for wear. If a band is worn or looks as if it could break, then replace it immediately.

In addition, there will also be considerations for sound equipment, microphones, instructor circuit cards, music tapes and any additional equipment such as skipping ropes, bean bags, boxing equipment, etc. that may be used in the aerobics room. Ongoing maintenance should be provided for all aerobic equipment. Consider storage and accessibility when planning to place equipment within the aerobics area.

Appendix I

The Travel Guide

Travel	Fwd	Bwd	Lat	OTS	Rotn	Comments
LIA Base moves						
Marching	✓✓	✓✓	X	✓✓	✓✓	
Step touch	✓✓	✓✓	✓✓	✓✓	✓✓	Zig-zag and/or fwd or bwd
Touch step	✓	✓	X	✓✓	✓✓	
Lift moves (see below)						
Variations						
Walk 1,2,3 touch	✓✓	✓✓	X	✓✓	✓✓	
Skipping	✓✓	✓	X	✓✓	✓✓	Caution: carpet footwear friction
Chasse	✓✓	✓✓	✓	✓	X	
Grapevine	✓✓	✓✓	✓✓	X	✓	Zig-zag fwd, bwd, str. fwd
Zorba	X	X	✓✓	X	✓	
Gallop	X	X	✓✓	X	✓	Sliding nature not suitable fwd or bwd
Low kick	✓	✓	X	✓✓	✓✓	
Knee lift	✓✓	✓	X	✓✓	✓✓	
Twisting	X	X	X	✓✓	X	Avoid twisting on carpet
HIA Base moves						
Running	✓✓	✓✓	X	✓✓	✓✓	
LIA jump/hop	X	X	✓	✓✓	✓✓	Lateral hops with knee lifts, etc.
Jumping	X	✓	X	✓✓	✓✓	
Variations						
Run hop (dbl run)	✓✓	✓✓	X	✓✓	✓✓	
Skipping	✓✓	✓	X	✓✓	✓✓	
Galloping	X	X	✓✓	X	✓	Caution with bwd galloping
Heels down	✓	✓✓	X	✓✓	✓✓	
Star jumps	X	✓✓	X	✓✓	✓✓	
Heel jacks	X	X	✓✓	X	✓	
Twisting	X	✓	✓	✓✓	✓✓	
Flick kicks	✓✓	✓✓	✓	✓✓	✓✓	Laterally one-legged
Knee lifts	✓	✓✓	✓	✓✓	✓✓	Laterally one-legged

Key: ✓✓ Good   ✓ OK   X Not successful

Appendix II

LOG-BOOK SUMMARY		
Type of class:		Date:
Fitness centre:		Time:
Equipment:		Tapes used:

Moves/exercises/choreography	Teaching method & learning curve	Organisation

Appendix III

Self-Test

The following 25 questions cover a range of topics from *The Aerobics Instructor's Handbook*. Use these questions as a self-test to gauge your knowledge both before and after you have read this book. Good luck! For most questions you will only need to answer true or false.

1.	A block in music adds up to 32 counts.	T/F
2.	The four high impact moves are running, jumping, lift moves and hi-squats.	T/F
3.	The hands-on method is the best way to correct a participant's form and technique.	T/F
4.	The EZQ system is a form of verbal communication.	T/F
5.	In a high impact class no more than 32 consecutive repetitions per foot strike patterns should be performed.	T/F
6.	When adding elements of variation, travelling and direction are classified as the same element.	T/F
7.	The Bare Bones stretch consists of a hamstring, compound pec and calf, hip flexor and lower back stretch.	T/F
8.	The 3 Ms of class preparation are: moves, music and motivation.	T/F
9.	The correct speed for Step is 118–128bpm.	T/F
10.	Pitch control may be used to increase music speed when attempting to increase intensity levels.	T/F
11.	The four hand positions to add the finishing touches to your movement are: the knife, fist, jazz and dance hands.	T/F
12.	If the class is performing an ezy walk with a right leg lead, you should lead with the left leg if in mirror image.	T/F
13.	When teaching choreography, the add-on method can be written A + B + C + D + E …	T/F
14.	A visual preview should be used when you are unable to break down and teach a combination.	T/F
15.	Linear progression, add-on and link are all common warm-up teaching methodologies.	T/F
16.	Two elements of variation include rhythm and mode.	T/F
17.	Complete the four directions of travel (****) on the aerobics compass at the bottom of the page.	
18.	A friendly body position is one in which you are crossing your arms.	T/F
19.	The 'When' in cueing refers to the name of the exercise that is to be performed .	T/F
20.	When receiving feedback from participants, it is recommended that you thank them.	T/F
21.	Relays are a form of organised action.	T/F
22.	Linear progression refers to changing one element at a time.	T/F
23.	Blitzing is a form of overload in muscle conditioning and involves working one muscle group or body part per track of music.	T/F
24.	The following movement sequence takes 32 counts to perform: (A) 2 x grapevines (R, L) + (B) 2 x ezy walks (R).	T/F
25.	Senior exercise groups consisting of semi-mobile and active mobile categories should use the rate of perceived exertion to measure intensity due to the effects on heart rate of medication, age and activity variations.	T/F

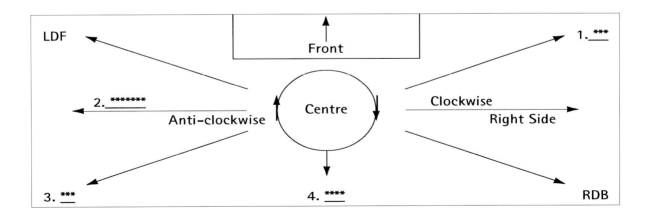

ANSWERS			
1. True	8. True	15. True	21. True
2. False	9. True	16. True	22. True
3. False	10. False	17. 1. RDF 2. Left side	23. True
4. False	11. False	3. LDB 4. Back	24. False
5. True	12. True	18. False	25. True
6. False	13. True	19. False	
7. True	14. False	20. True	

Glossary

1 Block	= 32 counts
1 Phrase	= 8 counts
ATT	Across the top
BPMs	Beats per minute
Bwd	Backwards
Cnts	Counts
CV	Cardiovascular
Dbl	Double
EZQ	Easy Cueing System
Fwd	Forwards
L	Left
Lead	Movement commences on that leg or foot
LLL	Left leg lead
OTS	On the spot
OTT	Over the top
R	Right
RLL	Right leg lead
ROM	Range of motion
RR	Rubberised resistance
Sgl	Single
Trail	Second leg or foot in the movement pattern

Bibliography

American Council on Exercise, *ACE Instructor Training Manual*, Chap. 14: 'Exercise and Pregnancy'.

American College of Obstetricians and Gynaecologists (ACOG), 1994, Guidelines for exercise in pregnancy and postpartum (Summary), bulletin no. 189, February.

American College of Sports Medicine, 1992, *Health/Fitness Facility Standards and Guidelines*, Human Kinetics Books.

American College of Sports Medicine Research Review, 1994, *Shape Fit Guide to Pregnancy*, Issue 1, Spring.

Oliver, K., 1997, 'Kids, the fun way to grow your membership', *Asiafit*, January/February, Hong Kong.

Pangallo, A., 1995, 'Voice Care', *Network News*, April/May, Australia.

Schwab, C., Levine S.R. & Crom, M.A., 1993, *The Leader in You*, Dale Carnegie & Associates Inc. Pocket Books, New York.

Index

Ability level, grading of 108
Accenting 34
Acknowledgement 59
Active mobile seniors 114, 115
Add and subtract method 44
Add-on method 43
Adjustments, technique 40
Aerobics class descriptions 104–107
Aerobics co-ordinator 110, 120
Aerobics facility, standards and guidelines 123
Aerobics room compass 32
Affective, learning 41
Agonist 79
Alignment, errors in 67
American College of Obstetricians and Gynaecologists 112
American College of Sports Medicine 113, 124
Anatomical breakdown 80
Antagonist 80
Appearance 57, 118
Armlines 9, 33, 34, 66
Auditions 122
Automatic, teaching process 40

Balance, teaching 40
Ballistic stretching 72
Bands 92
Barbell 87, 88
Bare bones stretch 65, 66, 74, 75
Base moves 8
   Aerobics 22-30
   Step 98–101
Basic comprehensive stretch 75
Basic regular stepping 96, 102
Beat 15
Beats per minute 19
Before class 58

Bilateral 31, 33
Block 16
Body language 38, 56
Body postures 56
Body Sculpt class 86, 107
Body weight resistance 78,
Bounce stretch 72
Breathing techniques 10, 88
Bridge 17
Bridge, advantages 18
Building rapport 57, 74

Cardio Funk 107
Carpet 124, 125
Cast offs 48
Circuits 46, 47
Children 77, 116
Choreography, teaching 7, 32
Chorus 17
Circles 49, 50
Class design 105
Class description 105-107
Class formats 93, 108
   Seniors 115
Class preparation 8, 58
Class introduction 55
Class standards and guidelines 125
Clothing 57, 118
Cognitive learning 41
Communication 54
   verbal 54
   non-verbal 56
Complexity 67, 109
Concentric contraction 80
Consecutive repetitions 42
Contact, points of 57
Continuing education 120
Contract-relax stretch 73
Compound movements 80
Contraindications, prenatal

exercises 113
Conversation 60
Cool-down 71
Core 80
Correction 40, 81
Count down, cueing 36
Cross-phasing 20
Cross training 106
Cueing 35, 81, 115
   What, When, Where, How 36

Demonstration 9, 38
Direction cueing 36
Direction 30
Double-ended relay 48
DR RT Lump 30
Dynamic stretching 65 72

Eccentric contraction 80
Education 60, 74
Educational cue cards 61
Elements of effective cueing 39
Elements of variation 30, 42
Employment issues 121
Entering a conversation 55
Equipment 86
   Storage 126
Evaluations 119
Exercise room 123
Exercise selection 38, 39, 87
Exercise vocabulary 9, 34
   Aerobics 22-30
   Muscle conditioning 81-82, 89-91, 93-95
   Step 98-101
EZQ system 36, 37, 38
Eye contact 56

Facial expressions 38
Facility 123

Feedback 119
Finishing touches 34
Fit facts 60
Fit Strips 92
Flexibility 72
Floor mix combinations, Step 102
Floor
    Space requirements 124
    Type and maintenance 124
Four-sided circuits 46
Four-sided triangle 46
Form and alignment 9, 79
Formations 11, 46–50
Funk 107

Gestures 56
Geographical cues 36
Getting the job 115
Goal setting 119
Grading 108, 109
Gravity 79, 89
Grip 88

Hand-held microphone 11
Hand positions 34
Handling situations 62
Hand weights 86
Heart rate 109
HIA, moves 26
Hi-Lo 105
Holding pattern 8, 18
    Addition 43
Humour 61

Imagery 82
Impact 22, 26
Incorrect speed 19
Instructing platform 125
Instructor
    Burnout 120
    Qualities 118
Instructor evaluations 119
Instructor positioning 11, 67
Instrumental 17
Intensity 31, 44, 71, 86, 109
Intermediate 109

Interval aerobics 106
Intonation 36
INTRO 55, 108
Interview 121
Isolation movement 80
Isometric contraction 80
Inverse stretch reflex 73

Kegel 114
KISS 40
Kids 77, 116

Layer Technique 44
Learning curve 41
Lever length 31, 87
LIA 22, 105
Light weights 86
Limitations of flexibility 72
Linear progression 42
Line circuits 47
Line of pull 79
Link method 43
Log book summary 8, 128
Loop 17
Lower body 80

Major positional exercises 81
Marketing 104
    Special populations 117
Microphone use 10
Mind wake-ups 62
Mirror imaging 11
Mix and match patterns 34
Mobility 65
Mode 31
Modern warm-up 64
Monitoring intensity 109
Moves 8, 22
Motivation 8, 58
Multi-peak 108
Muscle balance 79, 81
Muscle bulk 79
Muscle conditioning
    Class 93, 107
    Terms 79
    Step 103

Myths/misinformation 79
Muscular strength, power,
    endurance 80
Music 8, 15, 38
Music mapping 17
Music speeds 19, 66, 86
Music selection 15, 66, 73
Music volume 10, 21

Negative reps 84
Neutral footing 13
New Body 106, 107
New exercisers 53, 58, 68
Non-impact 29
Non-verbal communication 56
Non-verbal cueing 38
Novelty and themes 50

Omni-directional 10
On the top mixes, Step 102
Open position 56
Organised action 41, 45–51
On-the-spot (OTS) 31, 69
Overhead armlines 66
Overload 84

Pain and gain 79
Participant image 11
Participant expectations 120
Perceived exertion 109
Perimeter groups 46
Personal contact 57
Personal space 57
Phrasing 15
Pitch control 19
Plane 31
PNF stretching 73
Points of contact 57
Posture 9, 88
Power moves, step 103
Power words 102
Praise 59
Pre-adolescence 116
Pre-choreography 51
Pre-chorus 17
Pre-exhaustion 85

Pregnancy 77, 112
Preparation for classes 8, 35
Prenatal exercise classes 113
Principals of overload 84
Professional appearance 57, 118
Progressive relaxation 73
Prone 82, 83
Propulsion, step 103
Push Pull method 85
Pyramid method 42, 84

Qualities 118

Range of movement/motion
   (ROM) 65, 72, 85
Ranges of personal space 57
Rapport 35, 57
Recall 8
Recovery 71
Relays 47-48
Relaxation 73
Repetition 31
Reply to advertisement 121
Resistive exercise 78, 80, 86
Résumé 121
Reverse pyramid 42, 84
Rhythm 31
Rhythmic comprehensive stretch
   76
Ricochet 70
Right and left balance 43, 70
Right footing/arming 12
Rotational 31, 73
Rubberised resistance 92

Self-awareness 40
Self-test 129

Semi-mobile seniors 114, 115
Seniors 77, 114
Shape system 32
Side lying 81, 82
Single peak 108
Signage 126
Signs and symbols 38
Situations and solutions 62
Snakes 50
Sound equipment 20, 125
Specialty cool downs 77
Specific stretching 65, 77
Spirals 50
Spot reduction 61, 79
Standardise 36
Static stretch 65, 72
Starting/finishing positions,
   armlines 33
Staying motivated 120
Step 16, 96
   Class description 104, 105
   Safety guidelines 96
   Height 98
Storage, equipment 126
Stretches
   Essential 74
Stretch positions 67
Stretch reflex 72
Stretch variations 75-76
Stylised workouts 69
Super set 85
Supine 81, 82
Syncopation 34

Talk test 109
Tap free choreography, Step 102
Teaching choreography 41, 52

Teaching image 11
Teaching method, technique 41
Technical skills 7
The company, employment 121
Timetabling 110, 111, 121
Tone 80, 86
Top 'n' tail 44
Touching for rapport 57
Transitions 33, 42, 88
   Step 102
Travel 31
Trimester 112
Tubing 92

Unilateral 31, 33
Upper body 80

Verbal communication 54
Verbal cueing 36
Verse 17
Visual cueing 35
Visual previewing 39
Visibility 39
Vocal care 10
Voice projection 9, 40

Warm ups 64
   Specific 68
   Methodologies 69
Weighted workouts 68
Well timed cues 39
What to wear, interview 122
Wooden surface 124, 125
Workshops 8, 120

Zig-zag method 42, 69

Also available from Kangaroo Press

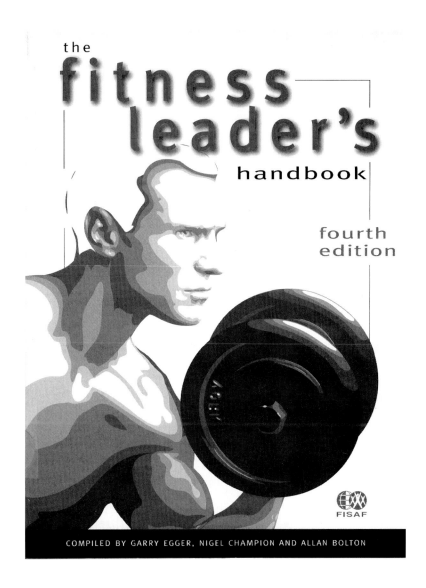

Fitness has become a way of life for a great many people. While numerous books have been written on the topic, few have detailed the scientific facts about exercise in an interesting, readable format. *The Fitness Leader's Handbook* does just that. This is the fourth edition, which has been thoroughly revised after nine years of extensive use.

The Fitness Leader's Handbook originated from lecture notes for the highly popular Fitness Instructor Training Program that has been conducted in Australia, New Zealand and many Southeast Asian countries. It provides up-to-date exercise prescription information for fitness instructors, school teachers, sports coaches, health professionals and anyone with a keen desire to improve their fitness.

The Fitness Leader's Handbook is the complete book of fitness and exercise programming. It is a useful addition to any home library and a must for any health professional.